P9-BYH-041

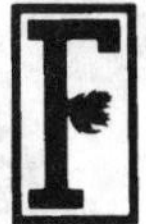

Hold

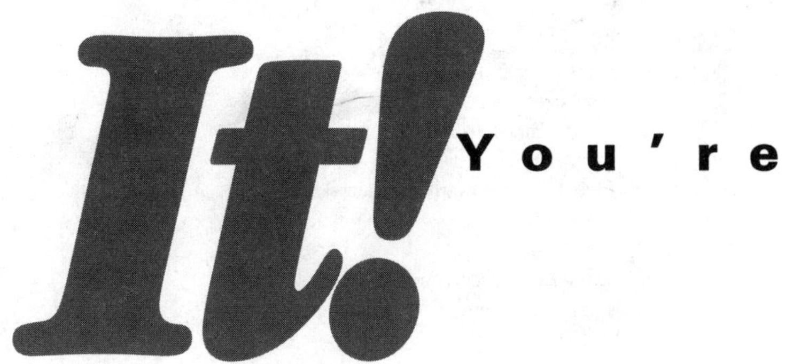

Hold It! You're Exercising Wrong

Edward J. Jackowski

A Fireside Book Published by Simon & Schuster
New York London Toronto Sydney Tokyo Singapore

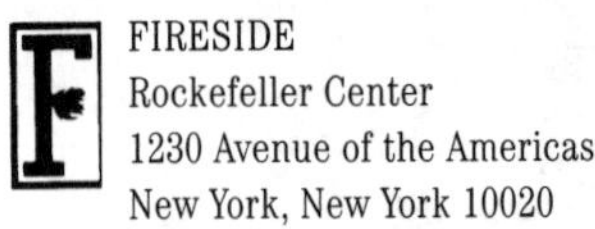

FIRESIDE
Rockefeller Center
1230 Avenue of the Americas
New York, New York 10020

Designed by Bonni Leon
Illustrations by Jerry O'Brien

Manufactured in the United States of America

10 9 8

Library of Congress Cataloging-in-Publication Data
Jackowski, Edward J.
Hold it! You're exercising wrong / Edward J. Jackowski.
p. cm.
"A Fireside book."
Includes index.
1. Exercise. 2. Physical fitness. I. Title.
II. Title: Hold it!
GV481.J33 1996
613.7'1—dc20 94-22719
CIP

ISBN: 0-671-89077-8

This publication does not reflect the views of the publisher. This publication contains the opinions and ideas of its author and is designed to provide useful advice in regard to the subject matter covered. Statements made by the author regarding exercise or the use of exercise equipment are based on the author's research and do not constitute an endorsement of any particular exercise product by the publisher. The publisher specifically disclaims any responsibility for any liability, loss, or risk, personal or otherwise, which is incurred as a consequence, directly or indirectly, of the use of any exercise equipment or exercise video listed on the order form.

To my parents, especially my mother—who *never* allowed me to come into the house before sundown, thus creating an easy path for me to remain active the rest of my life.

To Eve Barth, whose guidance and hard work have helped me tremendously.

Contents

Four

Five

Six

Seven

Eight

Nine

Ten

About the Author

Edward J. Jackowski is the founder and president of Exude Inc., the nation's largest motivational and one-on-one fitness company. A fifteen-year veteran of the fitness industry, Edward Jackowski brings keen knowledge and a unique perspective to the crowded exercise and fitness business, which has enabled him to stand out among his competitors. Headquartered in Manhattan, Exude is the only fitness company that custom-designs workouts for clients by body type.

He recently opened the country's first body-type center in Manhattan. With locations throughout the U.S.A., Exude services clients around the country and abroad with Edward's FastFitness routine. Edward Jackowski is sought by companies to empower people to become self-motivated to exercise and to lecture on successful sales techniques, stress and time management, and improving productivity and morale. His trademarked body types and methodology can also be found in health clubs, spas, and other fitness-related facilities.

In addition to writing a number of fitness articles for various magazines and newsletters, he has written a fitness booklet, hosted a syndicated radio program, and has designed thousands of fitness programs for people of all walks of life, including soldiers from the United States Army and a number of non-profit organizations. An avid sportsman and all-around athlete, he is a member of American College of Sports Medicine (ACSM), the International Dance & Exercise Association (IDEA), and is certified with the Aerobics & Fitness Association (AFAA), in both Aerobic and Fitness Training. Edward Jackowski holds a specialized degree (B.B.A.), in Organizational Behavioral Management from the Bernard M. Baruch Business College.

Look for Edward Jackowski's next fitness book due out in 1998 on motivation and exercising for your body type.

Introduction

Everyone can change his or her body through proper exercise. Let's face it, since we're all going to exercise, we might as well do it right. This book can be *your* source for separating fallacies from facts on the subject. Apply these tips, and you'll become more productive, not only in fitness but in every facet of your life.

Why do nine out of ten individuals who exercise and work out do it incorrectly? Many reasons. "Do you exercise?" I ask my clients when starting to design an individualized fitness program for them. "Oh yes, I play tennis and golf on the weekends and occasionally play tennis during the week when I have time," they reply. Let's clarify something right from the beginning: recreational tennis and golf are not exercise, per se. They are really leisure activities. In other words, you're doing it backward.

TIP 1

Don't try to get fit by being active. You can become more active only by becoming fit.

Too often people's misconception about tennis, golf, skiing, and other activities causes them injury because they are not fit before they go out and enthusiastically enter into these sports. Take the avid player who says he can play tennis for three hours without getting tired. Is he fit? Not necessarily, because when I ask him to try to touch his toes or jump rope for one minute, he can't. Only then does he finally realize that there's more to fitness than just putting in court time. As I tell my clients, I won't teach you how to hit a tennis ball, but I'll teach you how to get to that ball with speed, power, and agility and to hit it with the same strength shot after shot—now *that's* fitness.

TIP 2

Fitness is *your* ability to do whatever you ask your body to do.

In short, can you run a mile without having to recover for two days afterward? Do you have flexibility? Can you lift a ten-pound curl bar and do a series of upper body exercises for twenty to thirty repetitions without becoming fatigued? Can you jump rope for ten minutes or more?

Can you ride a stationary bike for fifteen minutes or more maintaining 90–120 rpm? Can you do twenty-five to fifty bent-knee sit-ups on a mat without locking your feet under a bed or bar? If you can answer yes to *all* of the above, then you are truly fit. (Of course if you are injured, or otherwise physically challenged, you should not or will not be able to do all of these activities, but you can still do lots of other exercises, if properly shown.) Clearly, fitness consists of many elements, which I'll address in detail in this book. The main reason people do not get fit is because they were never properly educated in the field of fitness and therefore may be working hard at the wrong thing.

Who am I? Why should you believe me rather than another fitness guru? Well to begin with, I'm the founder and CEO of the largest motivational and fitness company in the country, based in New York City. I teach people from all walks of life how to incorporate a sound fitness regimen into their daily life despite any constraint—physical or mental. During the last fourteen years I have seen and consulted with over 12,000 people—businessmen and businesswomen, mothers, mothers-to-be, physically challenged, athletes, fifty-plusers, children, professional athletes, former athletes, weight lifters, dancers, and executives who travel frequently and need a surefire traveling regimen.

I decided to write this book because I've seen definite trends among my clients. Most of the people I've met who were exercising regularly were not truly fit. Of the people who weren't exercising, all lacked the motivation to exercise and knowledge about *how* to exercise as well as how to fit it into their busy schedules. Interestingly, both groups were equally ignorant about many facets of fitness and getting fit.

I've educated thousands about how to exercise properly, safely, efficiently, and effectively. All have learned to become self-motivated to make exercise a part of their lifestyle for the rest of their lives. Anyone can go to a gym, a spa, or a fat-farm. But can you learn how to motivate yourself to make exercise a good, healthy habit, just like brushing your teeth, or saying thank you?

When you finish reading this book you will have that ability. This book is intended to shock you. I challenge you to realize that whatever you have or haven't been doing for fitness is most likely very wrong. This book also contradicts many professionals in the field of exercise and fitness.

Everyone has a theory about exercise. But the fact is, if you do not warm up first, then stretch, work out hard, and finally cool down, you might as well not even do it. You'll get some fitness benefits, but not as much as the person next to you who exercises in this exact order. In addition, there is *no one* machine or exercise that can get you fit in and of itself. But there is a way to get fit—a system if you will—by using minimal equipment if you exercise according to your body type as well as other factors. These factors constitute the genesis of this book.

TIP 3

The most important element in becoming and staying fit is *consistency.*

The *key* to being consistent with your exercise regimen is to develop a fitness program that you can perform in any environment. As you read on you'll be newly educated about the world of fitness, and motivated enough to keep up a consistent program.

Most studies of exercise and its effects on various parts of our bodies do not adequately represent everyone. There are too many factors to take into account while testing an individual to determine the exact benefits and hazards of exercise. Most theories on exercise and fitness are just that—proposed but unverified explanations. For example, during the 1980s high-impact exercise and aerobic dance classes were the new craze in fitness. Today, it has been scientifically proven that for most people, high-impact exercise can be damaging. Now the same medical evidence is being brought to the surface about the hazards of step classes. For the past fourteen years, *nothing* has changed about my theories on exercise, I've just refined them; in another couple of years, I'm confident that everything mentioned in this book will be scientifically and medically proven as well. A piece of fitness equipment does not guarantee fitness, but using that equipment with proper techniques, in combination with other exercises, will. That was the driving force for me to write this book, to separate once and for all fact from fiction regarding exercise and fitness.

After writing hundreds of fitness columns, articles, and a small booklet on fitness, I'm ready to fill the knowledge gap on motivation and exercise. This book should be your fitness bible. You might not like or even believe some items, phrases, or philosophies in it, but they are all true. I'm often asked in interviews to describe what I do. My answer: I create a path for people to exercise properly and consistently despite any constraint in their lives. It doesn't matter which exercise is the best if you cannot make fitness a habit. Worldwide we are missing the boat. Only when you have created an environment to incorporate proper fitness into your lifestyle will you ever be and stay fit.

In my travels across the country as a motivator, lecturer, and designer of fitness programs for individuals and companies, I have seen what improper exercise can do—nothing. I have also seen what proper exercise can do for an individual: it is by far the single most important factor in reaching any and all of your personal, professional, and health goals. It is the most powerful natural drug you can take. But as with any drug, too much can also be bad for you. Read on to find out which exercises work best for *you*.

Hold It!

You're Exercising Wrong

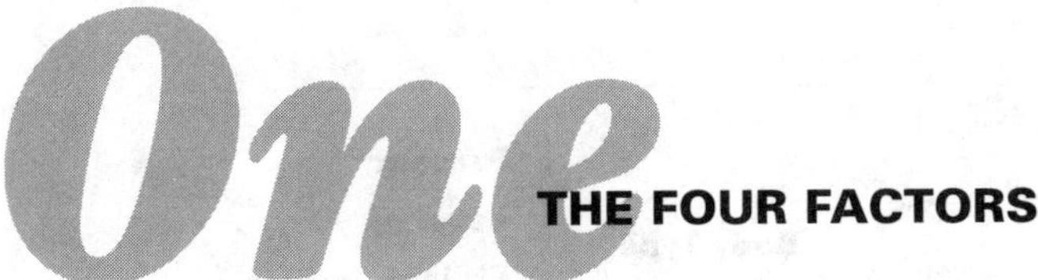

One

THE FOUR FACTORS TO CONSIDER WHEN STARTING OR MAINTAINING AN EXERCISE PROGRAM

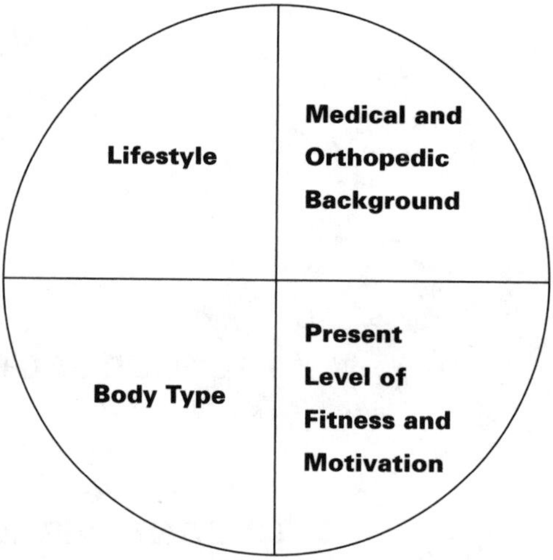

Lifestyle

Medical and Orthopedic Background

Body Type

Present Level of Fitness and Motivation

FOUR FACTORS CHART

LIFESTYLE

TIP 4

Your lifestyle dictates where and when you should exercise.

If you live in a city, there are certain kinds of stress you're going to encounter. If you live in the suburbs or on a farm, then you'll experience another kind of stress. Almost all stress is bad, except stress on the body from proper exercise. Why? Because stress equals strain. There is no such thing as "good" stress, nor are we that adept at controlling stress, let alone ridding ourselves of it. But we can control how stress affects our minds, bodies, and behavior.

TIP 5

You cannot relieve stress unless you exercise consistently and correctly.

One of the major fitness misconceptions comes from corporations and their so-called "stress management seminars." Human Resources directors will tell me, "We have a wellness program already in place." However, the fact is, you don't have a wellness program if your employees are not exercising on a regular basis at the workplace. Think about it: what good does it do to test employees for their cholesterol or blood pressure if you cannot directly help them lower it? These wellness programs are treating the symptoms, not the cause. Listen up, CEOs and other decision makers:

TIP 6

If your company does not have a *complete* in-house wellness program by the year 2000, every single profit will be eaten up in paying medical insurance for your employees.

Did you know that only two out of ten people who join health clubs go twice a week or more? You know why? Because they don't consider their lifestyle carefully before joining. Try to recall the last time you met with a health club or fitness company owner or salesperson. Did that person ever say, “Tell me about your lifestyle”? I probably would not have been as successful as I've been if health clubs, gyms, and spas didn't exist. Either people go and fail, or they join and don't go—then they come to me. Over 70 percent of my present and past clients have tried all of the above organizations to little, if any, success. But *they* did not fail, the system failed.

TIP 7

If only half of all your gym or club members showed up at the same time, the club wouldn't even be able to service half of the half that showed up. Why? Because they don't have the space or personnel to manage that massive number. Health clubs know that you won't show up, therefore they can sell, sell, sell.

Do you commute to work every day, travel often for work or leisure, keep long hours or work off hours, stay home with the children all day? Are you more than ten minutes' walking or driving distance from the nearest gym, afraid of sweating in front of others, feeling self-conscious exercising in front of others? If you answered yes to any of these then you just figured out *where* to exercise—at home. Remember, the most important factor in becoming and staying fit is *consistency.* If you can't be regular with exercise, it doesn't matter how great your exercise regimen is—you'll fail.

Now that you've figured out where to exercise, next you need to organize your day to find the time to do it.

TIP 8

If you're exercising for more than one hour, you're doing something wrong—unless, of course, you're training for a competitive sport.

Your entire workout (remember the four crucial phases: warming up, stretching, workload, and cool-down), which includes aerobic and anaerobic conditioning, does not need to exceed sixty minutes.

One of the most common mistakes people make with their exercise program is that they work out for hours, and then when they cannot find hours to work out, they don't do anything at all. This hurts in two areas. First, you can never achieve consistency. Second, if your body becomes used to exercising for hours and you have to cut down on time, you won't reap the benefits for that shorter period of time. The key is to be able to exercise under any time constraint.

When is the best time to exercise?

TIP 9

There is no scientific documentation that proves you get more benefit from exercise during the morning or afternoon.

The best time to exercise is when your schedule allows you to devote at least thirty minutes or more on a consistent basis. However, I have witnessed that when we perform aerobic exercises in the morning, our energy level is higher than when we perform strenuous anaerobic exercises in the morning. This is partially due to the fact that for most of us, our bodies are not fully alert and awake in the morning. Therefore, shocking our systems and raising our heart rate quickly, which is what happens when we perform anaerobic exercises, doesn't seem to be as effective at that hour.

TIP 10

Don't split up your exercise program throughout the day.

In other words, don't do sit-ups in the morning and jog at night. This takes us once again back to our formula—every time you exercise you must perform the four phases of every workout: warm-up, stretch, workload and cool-down. Otherwise, you might as well not even work out. By splitting the workout, neither outing would be completely productive, unless you follow the four phases.

MEDICAL AND ORTHOPEDIC BACKGROUND

You've heard it before and I'll reiterate it here: before beginning any exercise program, check with your doctor first. It is especially vital for certain individuals to get their doctor's approval prior to starting exercise: patients on heart medication, under an orthopedist's care, with a rare disease or unusual disorder, taking medications that affect the heart rate, or suffering from a bad back, just to name a few. More important than what to do is what not to do. This will ensure that you will not permanently injure yourself while attempting to exercise. Everybody, regardless of whether or not they presently exercise, should have a full physical and a stress test every year if they are thirty-five or older. Why? Because, if there is anything wrong with you, it will likely be detected during the physical and dealt with before it becomes severe. View exercise as a medication—a medication that is so powerful that it can positively change your overall well-being. Your medicine cabinet should have less pills, and your appointment book should have three to four red-inked exercise appointments in it per week.

TIP 11

If you don't find time for fitness, sooner or later you'll have to find time to stay home and be sick. What's a better business decision, to invest three hours a week in fitness or to miss a couple of days, weeks, or even months of work because you suffered a heart attack or some other ailment?

Everybody, regardless of age, present physical condition, or any physical constraint, can exercise. Your medical and orthopedic background will dictate the type of exercise you should be doing and the intensity level at which you should be doing it. Would you go out and try to run a mile in five minutes if you have not done so in ten years? Would you run a mile or jump rope or jump on a pogo stick if you had a slipped disc? Probably not. Common sense and good advice will guide you.

TIP 12

Regular and proper exercise can be the *key* to helping cure most ailments.

Unfortunately, because it requires effort, most people would rather take a magic pill because it's easier. Little do they know that the pill is really the long way to becoming healthier, whereas a good fitness program is the shortcut to being healthier in mind and body.

TIP 13

After engaging in a regular exercise program for one year, your body reacts as if you've been exercising your entire life. Remember, it's never too late to start!

Believe it or not, everyone can improve their physique *if* they learn to do specific exercises. Even spot reducing in those problem areas is possible thanks to my formula for exercising according to body type.

In fact, one of the main reasons I started my fitness company was because I had never met anyone who was totally happy with the way they looked, even though they exercised on a regular basis. For the past fourteen years, I have been perfecting the ultimate fitness system—a fitness program that will not only get people fit, but the *only* program in existence that effects change in one's body in as little as two weeks.

Body type is basically determined by genetics; however, certain factors influence how your body looks as you enter adulthood. Such factors include: how active you were growing up and are presently, your diet as a child and teenager, whether you exercise at all, and most important, the type of exercise you do for your particular body type.

TIP 14

A great diet can never make up for lack of exercise, but a great exercise program can make up for lack of a great diet.

Your body type is the pattern governing where and how your total weight is distributed—in other words, how much of your total body weight is carried on your upper body as opposed to your lower body. If you put on weight, where does it naturally go first?

TIP 15

Body type has nothing to do with how much fat or muscle your body has. It has nothing to do with whether you're fat, obese, thin, tall, short, athletic, or nonathletic. It simply means that if you added weight or lost weight, where on your body would that be most evident?

What's important to realize is that for your particular body type, certain exercises will help reshape your body to look better or worse. You can never change your body type, but you can dramatically change how your body looks *if* you understand how to exercise the right way.

Body types have traditionally been classified into three rather general categories: ectomorphs, which are lean and sinewy; endomorphs, which are bulkier; and mesomorphs, which are nearly perfectly symmetrical. I disagree with this system because I feel it does not truly describe and categorize every body.

The new names I've given the basic body types are easier to remember, but more important, because of their descriptive names, you'll understand what your body type is. I've identified four basic body types likened to devices that we either use, possess, or see in our everyday lives, and while we may easily identify with one of them, most people are actually a combination of types.

A *CONE*-shaped person has the following characteristics: Bigger on top, could even be top-heavy, has a tendency to add bulk from the waist up yet stays slim from the hips down. Like a cone, the top of his or her body is larger and as you move down the body, he or she becomes relatively more slender.

TIP 16

Cones need to make sure that their abdominal and pectoral muscles are very strong because of the excess weight that they carry in their upper bodies.

Heavy weights are a no-no for upper body exercises, particularly for women who don't want to build a bigger chest and torso. Although they are slimmer from the hips down, cone types might have a tendency to bulk up; if so, stair climbers, step exercises, squats, and heavy weights are not recommended. Very light weights and high repetitions for each exercise will do the trick. Running may be uncomfortable for cone types because of possible discomfort in the upper body; using a stationary bike is a good alternative for aerobic conditioning.

A *RULER*-shaped person carries the same proportion of weight on the upper as the lower part of the body and does not have a lot of curves. (An overweight person can still be ruler shaped if his or her weight is distributed equally.) There is not a very big difference between the size of your hips and the width of your shoulders, or the size of your upper body compared to your waist—like a ruler, you have virtually no difference in size between top and bottom. Generally, a woman ruler has small to medium size hips, almost like a boy's—in fact, ruler-type women make up the majority of fashion runway models.

TIP 17

Rulers possess the perfect body type to run, do stair climbing, and utilize heavier weights because they do not bulk up as fast, and it is usually very hard for them to add mass or size. And if they do, it's just as easy to add size to their upper body as to their lower body, or to lose mass in their upper as well as lower body.

The *SPOON* body type is typically reserved for women. The spoon's handle represents the top half or upper body, then at the base or lower part of her body she widens out. Sometimes when we look at a woman with this body type, we tend to think she is heavier than she actually is, because there is a noticeable difference between her upper and lower body. Spoon types have a tendency to bulk up or add mass to their lower body, yet their upper body does not gain size as easily. For the lower body, stair climbers, steps, squats, heavy weights, and stationary biking with a lot of resistance or tension is bad news. Although you'll become firmer, you'll push the fat on your body out farther and farther.

TIP 18

For spoon types, jumping rope and stationary biking at a very high speed with low tension or resistance are ideal for your lower body.

Also essential for reducing your lower body are calisthenics on a mat—without ankle weights. Your upper body is generally much weaker and therefore can use some resistance work, but be careful, because even though you are smaller on top you may have a tendency to bulk up a bit on your upper body.

Finally, the *HOURGLASS*-shaped person is also most likely a woman. This body type is solid and thick in both the upper and lower body. Don't despair! Although you have a tendency to bulk up or add mass and size easily, you can also lose that mass and size in proportion. Just as the ruler-shaped body can add size proportionally, you can lose that mass proportionally. You may be unhappy about having a body type like this, but believe it or not, with this particular shape it is easier and faster to obtain visible results if you exercise correctly. You have to be very careful not to bulk up your body, though, because hourglasses add size faster to the entire body than any other body type.

It is a lot easier to lose mass and size than it is to add size to one's body, since it takes a lot more time to add size, and you constantly need to be eating more which doesn't work for most people's lifestyles.

Stay away from these exercises if you are hourglass-shaped: stair climbers, steps, all heavy weights, squats, lunges, leg presses, aerobics classes, and running with or without weights in your hands. Exercises to do: jumping rope, stationary biking at a light tension, calisthenics, and a light curl bar routine for your upper body.

Summary

What's important to remember about all body types is that no matter what type you were born with, *everyone* can improve how they look. What's also important is not to "think thin," but to concentrate and work toward becoming slender for your body type.

OVERVIEW OF BODY TYPES

Cone®

Characteristics

bigger on top
tendency to add weight or muscle mass on top half of body
slimmer from hips down

1. Exercises to avoid:
heavy weights for upper body
rowing machine
jogging with hand weights

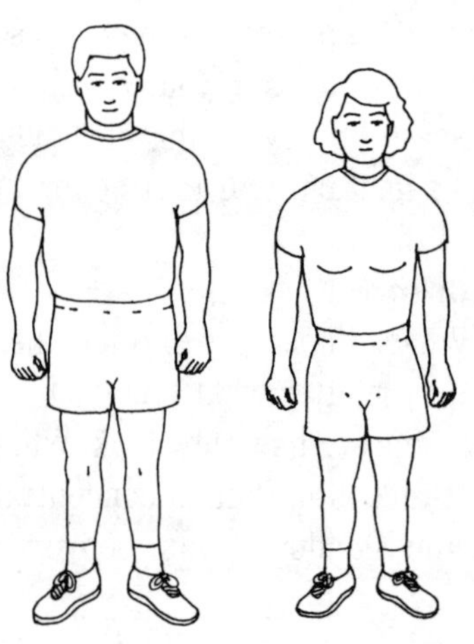

2. Borderline exercises:
running
stair climbers
jumping rope
aerobic dance
swimming
racquet sports

3. Recommended exercises:
light weights for upper body, high repetitions
stationary bike, moderate to high tension
leg exercises, moderate weights
abdominal exercises on exercise mat
good mornings
stair climbing—if you bulk easily

Ruler®
Characteristics

equal body proportions
weight gain distributed evenly on the body
weight lost evenly as opposed to one main area
often have small to medium-sized hips

1. Exercises to avoid:

None, providing you are orthopedically sound and are not very overweight

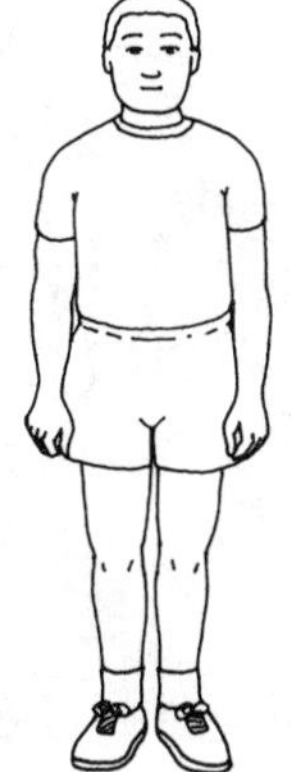

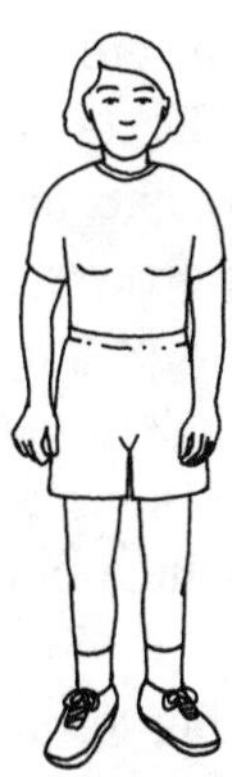

2. Exercises to avoid if you are very overweight:

heavy weights
stationary bike with moderate to heavy tension
squats with weights
stair climber
step classes

3. Recommended exercises:

running
jumping rope
stair climber
step aerobics
moderate weights for upper and lower body
stationary bike with low to medium tension
aerobic dance
swimming
rowing machine
calisthenics

Spoon®
Characteristics

upper body relatively smaller and weaker
tendency to bulk on lower half from weight gain or working with weights
difficult to lose weight and mass from lower half
fat on outside of thighs difficult to get rid of

1. Exercises to avoid:
stair climber
step aerobics
moderate to heavy weights for lower body
leg presses/squats
stationary bike with moderate to heavy tension
jogging/running

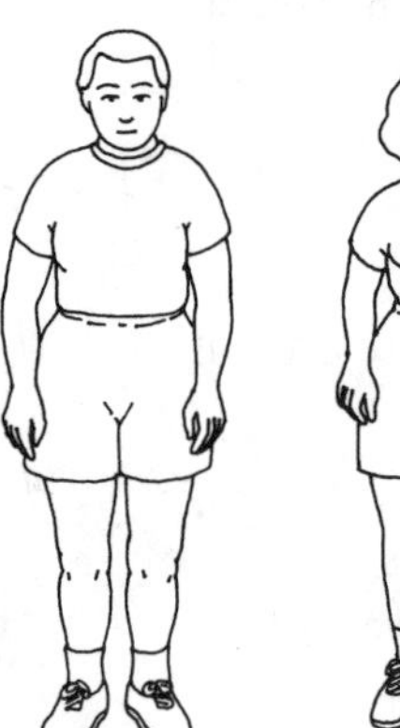

2. Borderline exercises:
walking
rowing machine
lunges

3. Recommended exercises:
jumping rope
stationary bike with low resistance
moderate to heavy weights for upper body
light weights for lower body, high repetitions
calisthenics on exercise mat
vertical scissors
standing knee to opposite chest with aerobic bar

Hourglass®
Characteristics

bulk or lose weight easily throughout entire body
tend to be solid in both upper and lower body
tend to be a little more slender through waist
body is otherwise proportional

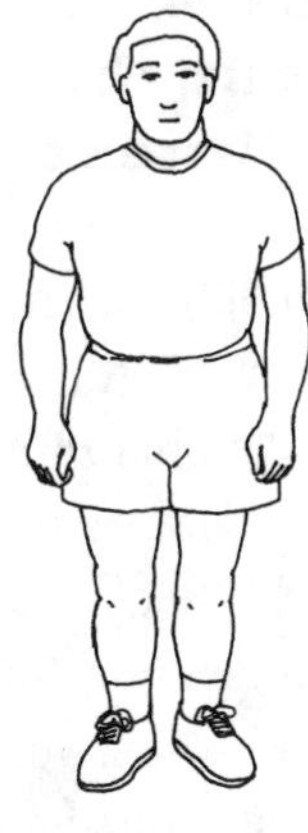

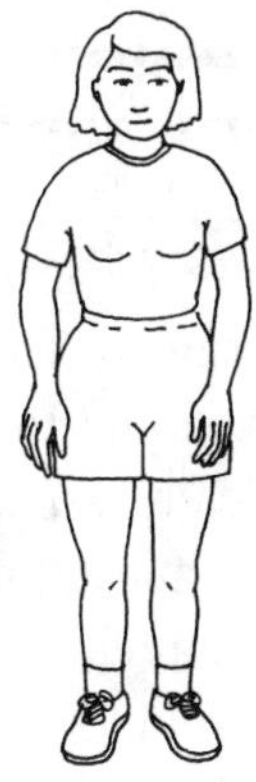

1. Exercises to avoid:
stair climbers
step aerobics
all heavy weights—for both upper and lower body
squats
lunges
leg presses

2. Borderline exercises:
walking
swimming
jogging/running

3. Recommended exercises:
jumping rope
stationary bike, light tension
calisthenics
5–10 lb. curl bar routine
stomach, leg, and hip routine on mat

TIP 20

The only way to become more motivated to exercise is to educate yourself about the different aspects of fitness.

I'm always amazed after spending an hour with a client and they turn to me and say, "Edward, just write down what we did today, and I'll be able to do it on my own." I typically respond, "If I came to work in your office for an hour, and afterward you decided to take a two-week vacation, could you go away feeling totally confident that I could run your business effectively? I hardly think so." When you word it like that it hits home, doesn't it?

How can you further educate yourself about fitness? Read magazines, health newsletters, and attend fitness seminars. Try to read both consumer and trade publications on fitness and exercise. *(IDEA, Fitness Management, American Journal of Health Promotion, Prevention, Men's Health,* and *American Fitness* are good ones.) To get ahold of the trade publications contact your local fitness center, which should have subscriptions and information to give you. Do not limit yourself to only reading fashion magazines for information on lifestyle and fitness. Only a handful of the beauty and fitness editors are as well versed on the subject as they should be.

TIP 21

Whatever you do, do not ask a friend for advice unless, of course, he or she is an expert in the field.

There is a lot of confusion as to who is an expert in this industry and who is not. I expect experts in *any* field to have the following criteria: they have spent a minimum of ten years in their chosen profession, have specialized in only a few areas of that field, have gotten proven, consistent results over a period of time, and, most important, have hands-on practical experience in that particular field.

Unfortunately, I would say that on a scale of one to ten, 99 percent of the so-called experts in the fitness field rate about a 2. I can say that with conviction because 90 percent of my clients have tried these "experts" and their theories on exercise, yet failed. People always ask me what's so unique about my program. I answer simply, (1) it works; (2) regardless of the environment you find yourself in, you'll be motivated and educated to maintain your fitness regimen for the rest of your life; and (3) it's the safest, most efficient, and most effective exercise methodology in the world today.

Everyone is searching for a way to become self-motivated to exercise.

I'm an expert in motivating you to incorporate fitness into your life, for the rest of your life. In addition, I've been fortunate enough to invent a fitness methodology that is more effective than *anything* in existence. Do you know what a thrill it is to see a person's body change in two weeks? Do you realize the power and confidence that this individual now possesses for the rest of his or her life! This is especially rewarding when he or she has been working out for the last couple of years with little or no visual results.

Unfortunately, the education and motivation you will receive from a club, gym, or spa is often wrong. Their instructors are not experts in designing lifestyle and fitness programs. Most of them are experts in designing a fitness program based on the equipment that the facility has on their premises. There is a big difference between putting someone on a machine, teaching him or her how to use it, as opposed to educating that same person about whether or not they even need to be using that machine.

TIP 23

Whether you're just starting out with exercise or are exercising regularly, it's important to decide how complex your fitness program should be.

If you travel often, you do not want to be exercising with a lot of fancy machines, because while you're away, you will not be able to keep up with it. Most people who travel frequently say they'll get back in shape when they return. They fall into the same pattern as a yo-yo dieter.

Finally, look in your local yellow pages for companies or individuals under the heading "Exercise Programs." Typically, they are more in tune with what you may or may not need. Also, speak to doctors, physical therapists, exercise physiologists, or chiropractors who use exercise as a form of rehabilitation. Ask to speak to some of their current or past clients to see if their own personal goals were achieved with the help of these individuals. And remember, when starting or maintaining a fitness program, do not attempt *any* exercise you are not familiar with, without proper supervision.

Two

THE ABC'S OF EXERCISE

PERCEPTIONS ON EXERCISE

Everyone can make a positive change in the way they look, feel, and perceive themselves if they learn to incorporate a safe, efficient, and effective exercise program into their daily life.

To many, *exercise* is still a dirty word because they feel they have to force themselves to do it. Another reason people are uneasy about fitness is that they are uncomfortable with the process of becoming regular with their fitness program. When we get overworked with stress, exercise is usually the first thing we stop doing. What we don't realize is that exercise is an extremely powerful tool to help us through that stressful period. Time constraints should not be an excuse to skip workouts; in fact, your exercise program should be time efficient.

To succeed in whatever you choose to do with your life, you need five key ingredients: focus, discipline, persistence, product or service knowledge, and talent. Exercise acts as a catalyst in providing the energy necessary to maintain these five elements. If exercise is sacrificed, then it becomes difficult to achieve success in other endeavors. These are the top five excuses I consistently hear for not working out:

1. Not enough time
2. Not motivated
3. Don't like it
4. Never see results
5. Physical constraint (bad back, obesity, pregnancy, bad knees)

What do all these excuses have in common? They're *perceived* constraints. When you go to the refrigerator to get something to eat, do you negotiate with yourself and ask "Should I open it?" When you're ready for bed, do you stand by the bed and ask "Should I lie down to rest?" When you brush your teeth, do you even have to think about it? The same is true when you sit down to relax and watch television or read. Then why then do we have to negotiate with ourselves when it comes to exercise? Because we haven't made it a habit. When we are able to make exercise become a habit in our lives, then it will require less thought. Try to make fitness a part of you. Everybody needs exercise.

TIP 24

Only a fit person can work and play with vigor and enthusiasm. Vitality and relaxation are enhanced by being in good physical condition.

THE PHYSICAL AND MENTAL BENEFITS OF FITNESS

The fitter you are, the more your body and mind can withstand fatigue. A fit individual has a stronger and more efficient heart and can tolerate stress more effectively. In fact, there is a definite relationship between mental alertness, absence of nervous tension, and physical fitness.

TIP 25

The next time you come home from work feeling tired and you do not have enough time to take a short nap, get on that stationary bike or treadmill for twenty minutes. Break a sweat, and before you know it, you'll feel totally revived!

Levels of physical and mental fitness are different for everyone. Unfortunately, though, very few people know how to best judge what their optimum levels of fitness are or how to go about getting there. Very few people are fully in tune with their bodies or able to distinguish mental from physical fatigue.

TIP 26

Exercise can be a sedative for those who need to relax. And yet, exercise can act as an "upper" for those who are feeling sluggish or lethargic. Exercise is the most powerful natural drug known to mankind.

Nothing can alter your state of mind and body in a positive manner better than proper exercise. But like anything, too much of this good thing can also be hazardous.

TIP 27

Be careful not to overexercise, because if you do, you can suffer from insomnia, depression, and a feeling of constant fatigue.

People with low fitness levels often experience high levels of anxiety, fear, and depression. One of the fastest ways to gain control of your life is to ease your way into a fitness program and watch the positive results. Adopting healthy behaviors gives you the confidence to become more active in life. Many people reject exercise because they are not confident they can achieve fitness, or they feel rejected by fit and active people as a result of their poor fitness level.

Remember high school gym class, where either you or one of your fellow schoolmates were always chosen last when picking teams? Although it is definitely true that some people are blessed with more athletic ability than others, we can all vastly improve our athleticism with proper instruction and perseverance.

TIP 28

***Everyone* can become a better athlete if taught the fundamentals of fitness.**

I remember trying to get a successful attorney on a fitness program. He would not return my phone calls for five months. Finally I got him on the phone and said to him, "Give me eight minutes, and I'll change your life." Today, he is fit and we are the closest of friends!

He had been exercising six days a week for the previous ten years and had no agility or coordination and, worst of all, no self-confidence, especially when it came to playing sports. I taught him that if shown how to perform an exercise correctly, he could master it with time and practice. I taught him to jump rope. He did it. I just provided the motivation and gave him the confidence. I convinced him that if he persevered as he did in law school to become a top attorney, he could also become great at using his body. The key is that after spending time disciplining himself and working on his weak points, that feeling of accomplishment carried over into every other facet of his life, personally and professionally. This man has been transformed into a strong, confident, and more secure person.

TIP 29

Use exercise to cleanse your mind and emotions. If your mind is cluttered, it will become fresh following exercise.

If you're exercising properly, it is the only time that your mind actually rests. Even when we sleep, our brain works. That's why out of all the people I've interviewed who exercise regularly, those who work out at home, where they can pay attention, are not only more fit but much more productive. I'm not against health clubs or gyms, but if you're distracted by anything else besides fitness while exercising, you will not reap all the benefits that come with fitness.

TIP 30

You cannot relieve stress and get the full benefit of exercise if you're in an environment where you are constantly being physically, mentally, and sexually stimulated.

If you find yourself not being able to concentrate and work out in your present health club or gym, consider exercising at home three days a week. Go to the gym on your off days when you just want to jog leisurely on the treadmill or ride the stationary bike.

TIP 31

The benefits you derive from your exercise will grow as your fitness level increases.

THE *REAL* PHYSICAL AND MENTAL BENEFITS OF FITNESS:

If you *don't* exercise, you will not have: energy, self-confidence, a good night's sleep, a firm and toned body, an outlet for stress, a strong back, a fulfilling sex life, strong bones, a strong heart, low LDL cholesterol, a strong aerobic capacity, good circulation, rosy cheeks, the ability to handle stressful situations, an active lifestyle, healthy friends, new hobbies, good posture, frequent desserts, a clear perspective on ideas, issues, problems and solutions, new challenges, the ability to relax, a positive outlook on life, the ability to be a good loser.

If you are smart and do exercise, you will have: energy, self-confidence, a good night's sleep, a firm and toned body, an outlet for stress, a strong back, a fulfilling sex life, strong bones, a strong heart, low LDL cholesterol, a strong aerobic capacity, good circulation, rosy cheeks, the ability to handle stressful situations, an active lifestyle, healthy friends, new hobbies, good posture, frequent desserts, a clear perspective on ideas, issues, problems and solutions, new challenges, the ability to relax, a positive outlook on life, the ability to be a good loser.

One of the most difficult skills to develop is the ability to differentiate between the excuses for why you don't exercise and the real reason(s) why you don't. Is the fear due to lack of education about exercise? Are you lazy? Do you have a medical condition that you don't want to aggravate further? Whatever the reason, be honest with yourself and speak to an experienced motivation and fitness expert to help overcome that obstacle.

TIP 32

There is a direct correlation between educating yourself on fitness and your motivation to keep it up.

Training yourself to *want* to exercise is the key. However, it takes time to make exercise a part of your regular routine. How do we train ourselves to want to exercise? A surefire way to help motivate ourselves and to keep motivated to make fitness a regular part of life is to see quick results. That's why it's imperative not to just exercise but to exercise properly.

TIP 33

Just because you're exercising, doesn't mean you are getting fit.

Exercising regularly will entice and excite you to keep on with your lifestyle change. Education is the *key* to motivation. As you learn more about fitness and which exercises are best for your body type, you will improve your fitness level and self-motivation.

Time constraints are a major reason why people fail to keep up with their exercise programs. It's easy to become dependent on certain classes, trainers, instructors, and equipment that are available at specific times. Try to structure your fitness program so that you're not solely dependent on these extraneous factors.

TIP 34

Don't rely on a buddy for fitness, because if you do, when he or she does not show up, most likely you won't go through with your workout either.

If you have a number of different fitness routines—a long workout and a mini workout routine—you'll never miss a workout because of time constraints.

TIP 35

Do not rely solely on exercise classes, because if you cannot make it on time, you'll find yourself skipping workouts completely. Have an alternate routine for those days when you can't make your regular class.

We all know that we need to exercise, but why does only 20 percent of the American population exercise two to three times per week? And out of that 20 percent, only 1 percent do it correctly! We need to make fitness a *priority.*

Take action! Align yourself with people you know who are active, or be a spectator at a local athletic event. Take note of the grace and athleticism involved in these sports. Also, open your appointment book and schedule your first meeting with a lifestyle expert, someone who specializes in custom-designing fitness programs. This person will provide the initial motivation and demonstrate how you can realize your fitness goals.

THE FOUR ESSENTIAL PHASES OF EVERY WORKOUT

Before you read on, let me state emphatically that if you do not follow the exact order of these four phases every time you exercise, then you will *not* gain the true benefits of fitness, hence you'll never be fit!

Phase I: The Warm-up

Warming up is *not* stretching. Often I hear, "Did you stretch?" "Yeah, I warmed up." Or, "Did you warm up?" "Yes, I stretched." Warming up has many purposes: it provides a smooth transition from the resting state to the higher level of energy expenditure and effort you experience in the main part of your workout; it raises your heart rate from its resting state gradually and safely in order to prepare your heart for more demanding activity. It prepares the body physiologically and psychologically for physical performance, not only to improve performance but also to lessen the possibility of injury.

TIP 36

A proper warm-up will prevent and/or reduce strains and muscle pulls, tears, and soreness.

Warming up raises both the general body and the deep muscle temperatures and stretches collagenous tissues, which permits greater flexibility. It also increases your physical working capacity during your workout.

TIP 37

The time needed for satisfactory warm-up varies from individual to individual and tends to increase with age.

I recommend from five to fifteen minutes of warming up, depending on how fast your body takes to feel loose and break a steady sweat. The colder the weather, the longer your warm-up should be. General warm-up procedures should consist of jogging, easy running, stationary biking, rowing, or other light aerobic activity. It should be of sufficient duration and intensity without developing marked fatigue.

The nature of the warm-up varies to some degree in relation to the activity. For instance, if you are a long distance runner, try to warm up by jogging at a slow pace for ten minutes rather than biking or rowing. You want to simulate as close as you can the physical activity you're about to engage in. Some warm-ups lend themselves well to athletic activities of all types; other warm-ups are specifically designed for the sport in which you are participating. The best warm-up for most exercisers and sports enthusiasts is stationary biking with minimal resistance. I have found that it raises your heart rate more safely than treadmilling, for example, and it really loosens up your entire lower body as well.

TIP 38

No more than ten minutes should elapse between the completion of the warm-up and performing your exercises.

Phase II: Stretching

Once warmed up, you can begin to stretch. This should take between four and seven minutes, depending upon your age and how flexible you are. As you age, you need more time to stretch your muscles.

TIP 39

You cannot increase body tone unless you increase your flexibility. That's why many people take an exercise or aerobics class for years without really changing their bodies.

Flexibility is one of the most important factors in increasing your fitness level. To some, flexibility comes easily; to others, it is the most uncomfortable part of working out. Quite often those who skip stretching do so because they are not good at it and do not realize its importance.

Certain types of exercises can either increase or decrease your flexibility. Jogging and running tend to tighten your hamstrings, and heavy weight lifting, unless properly performed, will decrease your overall flexibility.

So it is very important to make sure you're stretching. I have found that high-impact aerobic and step classes also decrease flexibility. For those who do a lot of stationary biking, you tend to have better hamstring flexibility but your quadriceps (tops of thighs) tend to be tighter.

TIP 40

Genetics do play a role in flexibility, but *everyone* can increase their flexibility if they learn the correct techniques.

I've never worked with anyone, regardless of age, who has not dramatically increased their flexibility within a short period of time. Stretching prepares the body for shock, for the physical demands you are about to put on your muscles.

Good flexibility increases your ability to avoid injury; since it permits a greater range of movement within your joints, the ligaments and other collagenous tissues are not so easily strained or torn. It also permits greater freedom of movement in all directions. Conversely, hyperflexibility must be avoided, because loose-jointed individuals are more prone to dislocations and other injuries. Extremes in flexibility are indeed of little value and can result in weakness of the joint at certain angles. Flexibility, like strength, is quite specific to the joint and its surrounding complementary tissues. It varies from one person to the next.

Stretching promotes circulation and feels good. The

correct way to stretch is a relaxed, sustained (static), stretch, concentrating on the muscles being stretched. The wrong way (unfortunately practiced by most) is to bounce up and down (ballistic), or to stretch until you feel pain, which can do more harm than good.

TIP 41

When you stretch, hold the stretch for ten to sixty seconds. Do this with each stretch. This is called *static* stretching.

Hold a static (nonmoving) stretch so that the specified joint is immobilized in a position that places the desired muscles and connective tissues passively at their greatest possible length. Little risk of injury exists if static stretching is performed.

Stretch until you feel a *mild* tension, and relax as you hold the stretch. The feeling of tension should subside as you hold the position. If it does not, ease off a bit and find a degree of tension that is comfortable. If you can, stretch slightly farther and continue to hold it. Again the tension should lessen; if not, ease off slightly. While stretching, breathe normally; exhale as you bend forward and continue breathing as you hold your stretch.

TIP 42

Do not hold your breath while stretching, and remember to relax your facial muscles.

If a stretch position prohibits your normal breathing, then you are obviously not relaxed. Ease up on the stretch in order to breathe more easily. In the beginning, silently count the seconds for each stretch. As you gain experience, you will be able to hold the stretch without counting and will hold each stretch by the way it feels. In chapter 10 you'll find an easy sequence of stretches to follow. Remember, stretching takes place only after the warm-up phase.

Phase III: The Workload

Now that you're properly warmed up and stretched, we can start the workload phase of your workout. As you can see, the first two phases of your exercise regimen are crucial, because they can protect you if you perform an exercise incorrectly. Most exercise-related injuries occur because of quick, jerky movements. Loosening up could prevent you from tearing a muscle or worse. We've all heard about people dropping dead while mowing a lawn or shoveling snow. You know why? These are examples of sudden exercise. If these people walked around the block a couple of times and did some light stretches before mowing or shoveling, it would probably save their lives. Remember, exercises that require short, quick movements are usually anaerobic in nature. Anaerobic-type exercises raise your heart rate very quickly, hence if your heart and muscles are not warmed up, the shock can cause a heart attack, no matter what activity or movement you are performing.

I recommend exercising three to six days a week, depending upon your goals, current medical condition, present fitness level, and any lifestyle constraints. Each workout should be designed so that you have a true understanding of what exercises are to be performed, as well as why and how you should do them.

TIP 43

To help individualize your fitness program and especially your workload phase, you must use the *REPS Principle.* Your body type is the most important factor in determining the sequence of elements within the REPS Principle. It will dictate which element comes first for your particular fitness program.

Here are the four elements that make up the REPS Principle:

Recurrence (R): The number of exercise sessions per week, that is, how many times per week you should repeat an exercise session.

Energy (E): Your energy is in direct relation to your intensity, or how hard you should work during each exercise session. The more intense your workouts become, the more energy is needed and used.

Period (P): How long each exercise period should be each time you work out.

Sort (S): What sort of exercises you should perform in order to effect positive changes in the way you look and feel.

TIP 44

By combining the four factors outlined in chapter 1—lifestyle, medical and orthopedic background, body type, present level of fitness and motivation—and following the REPS Principle, everyone can get and stay in top fitness form.

The REPS Principle applies equally to all people, but the sequence of elements within REPS changes depending upon their goals. For instance, the sequence for a person who wants to lose a lot of weight looks like this: RSPE. For a person who does not have weight to lose but whose goal is to firm up, the formula looks like this: SEPR. I will go into this in more detail in chapter 5 when we discuss how to get in shape and change your body according to your goals.

Phase IV: Cooling Down

Too often, because of time pressures, we tend to finish our aerobics class or weight training session and just leave the gym. Although it is difficult to persuade you to cool down your body after your workout, remember: you will not get the true benefits of exercising unless your body is sufficiently cooled down.

Cooling down refers to exercising at gradually diminishing intensity (energy) following strenuous work. It permits the return of both the circulation and other functions of the body to pre-exercise levels.

Most cardiac complications often occur with the cessation of exercise. A proper cooldown will continue to lower the heart rate and will also help to prevent excessive pooling of the blood in the lower extremities, reduce muscle soreness, and promote faster removal of metabolic wastes. The same way you warmed up your body to prepare for your workout, you must slow your body down after each workout.

TIP 45

Your energy output during your workout will dictate how long you should cool down.

I have found that riding a stationary bike or walking at a normal relaxed pace works best for cooldown. Your cool-down period, consisting of mild aerobic-type exercises, should range from four to eight minutes.

TIP 46

You know you're in good shape if, within five minutes of completing a vigorous workout, your heart rate falls to or below 100 beats per minute.

The cool-down period should not be as intense as your warm-up. It should be a notch or two lower in your energy output. Ride a stationary bike with little or no resistance (tension) until your breathing has returned to normal.

A lot of fitness enthusiasts stretch after their workout. There is conflicting evidence on whether or not stretching at the end of one's workout acts as an effective cooldown. I tend to think not. Stretching raises your heart rate from its resting state and does not lower it gradually. It is classified as passive recovery. However, what you need is active recovery, because it causes blood and muscle lactic acid levels to decrease more rapidly and keeps the muscle pumps going.

TIP 47

If you do want to stretch after your workout, cool down first, and remember to avoid overstretching, because certain muscles are fatigued and you're more susceptible to straining or pulling a muscle.

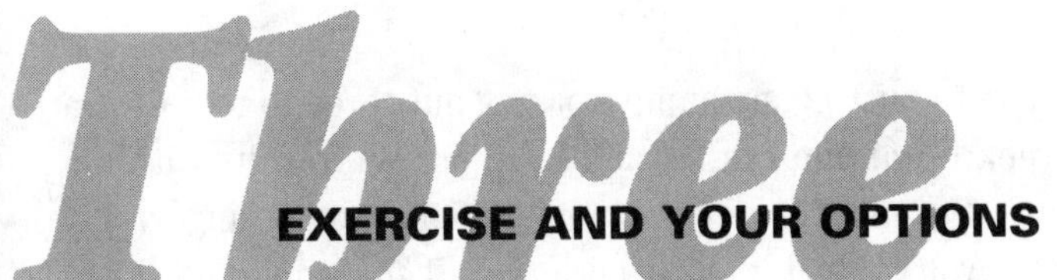

Three
EXERCISE AND YOUR OPTIONS

JUST BECAUSE YOU'RE EXERCISING DOESN'T MEAN YOU'RE GETTING FIT

If I were busting my hump working out three to four days a week for an hour or so, and I did not see results within a month, I would worry that I must be doing something wrong. Maybe you've had that experience. *What* could be going wrong?

Ask yourself: Did you follow the four phases that encompass every exercise session? If yes, are you exercising correctly for your body type? Do you have the right REPS formula? Now you see how many factors there are to consider when exercising. Fitness, though plausibly simple, has many facets. That's why you should not ask your friends how to exercise. Designing fitness programs is an art, a specialty, almost like that of a chef who prepares a gourmet meal. It's not that the chef adds any *one* special ingredient, it's the way he or she *combines* the ingredients, the order and type of spices, and knowing how long to cook it, that make it great.

The simple fact that you are exercising on a regular basis doesn't mean you are actually getting *all* the benefits—mental and physical—that can be gotten from exercise. Over the past twelve years, I have put thousands of clients through a fitness orientation. I would estimate that only 1 percent of these individuals were fit to begin with. In fact, some of those who made up the 1 percent were people who had hardly exercised at all. They just had good genes and had been athletes when they were younger. Although they did not pursue fitness on a regular basis, they were still very active in their jobs as well as on weekends.

Sometimes I consult with former or current professional athletes who are so unfit, it amazes me that they can make a living with their bodies. In comparing an unfit former athlete to an unfit nonathlete, I have found that the former athlete *always* gets into shape perhaps two to three times more quickly than the nonathletic person. An athlete is mentally tougher when it comes to fitness, because he or she has trained before and understands that in order to excel in any particular sport, it takes discipline, sacrifice, patience, and consistency. The nonathletes, who have never experienced this before, may not even know if they're fit yet and may find it more difficult to become in tune with their bodies. But great effort and dedication can pay off for an unathletic person. I've taught people who considered themselves uncoordinated to be very fit and athletic. Sure, it doesn't come as easy to all, but then, nothing does.

TIP 48

Persistence makes up for lack of skill in any endeavor you choose to master, especially when working toward your fitness goals.

Sometimes the lack of fitness among regular exercisers is shocking. Consider athletes who work out with heavy weights yet cannot perform simple upper body exercises with a fifteen-pound straight bar. Or people who do dozens of crunches in class, yet cannot perform ten perfect sit-ups. Or runners who run five miles a day, yet cannot jump rope nonstop for five minutes. Or how about all the aerobicizers taking all those exercise classes and not looking any better than when they started them?

It's surprising how unfit this country is, yet we keep doing the same fitness routines year after year. It's not our fault, however, because most of our exercise and fitness techniques come from supposed fitness professionals, and most of their exercise techniques are outdated. That's why it's important to keep up with advances in fitness, as well as to make sure we are working out in a way that will be most beneficial to our body types. As I always say to my clients: if you are going to go to the trouble of exercising, you might as well improve your body and your fitness level at the same time.

WALKING, JOGGING, SWIMMING, AND OTHER POPULAR EXERCISES

Walking

TIP 49

You could walk from New York to California and still not be fit.

Do you know anyone who walks for fitness whose body looks good and is fit? Remember the four phases of every workout? Even if you walk, you still need to warm up, then stretch, walk vigorously, and cool down. Walking by itself will *never* get you fit.

Here's why: walking puts undue stress on your back and knees; it tightens your hamstrings and other leg muscles; it can cause foot problems and ankle problems; it does nothing to increase your upper body strength; it does very little to strengthen your abdominals; it does very little to increase your agility, balance, coordination; and it does little to increase your strength and muscle endurance. If you do not have access to a treadmill, walking is weather dependent; if you live in a city, you have to worry about crime, noise, traffic, and other city constraints. Besides, walking does not increase your cardiovascular conditioning as effectively as other exercises; and it takes so much time to see results.

So why the great craze for walking? It's not expensive, no equipment is needed except for a good pair of walking shoes, and it does not require a lot of effort. I view walking as a leisure activity. Walk for fun, not for fitness. Exercise so that you can enjoy walking. Walking to and from work daily can add slight benefits to your cardiovascular health. Engage in your regular fitness program and use walking as a supplement.

Where does walking fit into your exercise program? Well, if you do not have access to any fitness equipment; it is an okay way to start an exercise program, provided you follow the four phases. Make sure, though, that you are walking fast enough to get your heart rate up in order to realize some physical benefits.

TIP 50

Walking, by itself, is not a complete fitness program.

Jogging

Jogging (running) can be more effective than walking, provided that you are orthopedically sound.

TIP 51

Jogging can put an enormous stress on your knees and back, and for most runners, it will tighten the hamstrings.

Many runners injure their feet from the pounding they endure on pavement. You might not feel pain in the beginning, but over time, everyone I know who runs has terrible feet, a bad back, and a very inflexible body. The other thing to consider when running is your body type. If you are big boned, heavyset, or vastly overweight, running is going to be much more difficult for you.

Take a look at your world-class marathon runners. How many of them weigh more than 160 lbs. for the men and 120 lbs. for the women? Also take a look at their body type—usually they're very slim, with narrow shoulders, small hips and thighs, and a very small upper body. Because of their slightness, they do not put a lot of stress on their joints when they run. But if you take a careful look at competitive runners, you will find that although they are slim, they are often still soft and flabby, especially around the middle.

TIP 52

Jogging is aerobic, and aerobic-type exercises take away mass but do not tone the body as much as anaerobic exercises.

On the flip side of the coin are sprinters. Their bodies are very muscular and very firm throughout. Sprinting is an anaerobic exercise. Sprinters are usually much broader throughout the shoulders, hips, and buttocks. Very rarely do you see a sprinter with the body type and muscle tone like that of a long-distance runner. So if you are naturally built like a sprinter, stay with sports that require short bursts of power and speed such as football, rugby, tennis, squash, basketball, volleyball, handball, and racquetball.

If you combine jogging or running with other forms of exercise, it can be a very effective way to get and stay in shape. But you should always have an alternate fitness routine, especially if you rely on running in a climate that makes you inconsistent. Remember, consistency is the most important element of a fitness program.

When starting to jog or run, make sure you ease into it. Start out by running about a mile. See how your body feels the next day or so. If you are very sore, do not increase your distance for a week or so. If you are not sore, then jack it up to two miles and see how your body reacts.

TIP 53

If you have a limited time budget, it is more beneficial to speed up than to increase distance. The more energy you put in, the more calories you'll burn and the fitter you will become.

One common mistake runners make is to keep running when they injure themselves. They think they can run it off, and yet years later they are diagnosed with stress fractures, slipped discs, and other problems.

TIP 54

When you injure yourself performing any exercise, you should rest that part of your body until it is almost 100% recovered.

If you want to engage in a jogging program, I suggest you read up on running and training techniques, so you can use the activity as an aspect of your fitness program. And, don't forget to stretch!

Swimming

If you have access to a pool on a regular basis, then I highly recommend swimming as a supplement to your fitness program. Swimming is very easy on your joints, and practically everyone of all ages can do it. It is also a very good way to rehabilitate most injuries, because the water offers resistance in every direction that you move your body. The problem is that people who choose swimming as part of their fitness regimen are not always consistent because of weather constraints, inconvenient location of the pool, and the time the workout takes. Also, swimming is one of the slowest ways to lose weight because it takes a lot of time to build up to swimming any distance. Usually people start out and swim a short distance (100 yards or so), stop and rest, then swim, then stop, etc. Consequently, swimming in the initial stages is anaerobic for most.

TIP 55

If losing weight is your goal, swimming is *not* the most effective and efficient way to go about it.

Rowing

Rowing is another good exercise, but the equipment is not the most manageable for in-home use. Also, not all gyms carry rowing machines. Rowing is an excellent exercise for increasing your cardiovascular capacity, but it tends to put some strain on your neck, shoulders, back, and arms. If you have a bad back or bad knees, then it is *not* the exercise for you. Rowing can be easier for men than women since most men have a naturally stronger upper body. Overall, it is a good way to get in shape if it does not put a lot of strain on your body.

Yoga

I know people who swear by yoga. Although I think yoga has advantages, it is still passive exercising. If you combine a sound fitness program with yoga, then it will add to your fitness level. But yoga alone will not get or keep you fit. It is also very time consuming. Besides, it is often hard to find qualified yoga instructors who really know what they are doing. When all is said and done, I think the benefits of yoga are more mind oriented than body oriented.

Ski Machines

Ski machines provide a very good aerobic exercise, but the equipment is typically costly. It's good to have an instructor help you at first, since it takes a great deal of coordination to perform the exercise properly. Initial difficulty often results in a loss of interest. Skiing is also very demanding on your cardiovascular system in the beginning, so you'll need to be taking lots of breaks. Some people have a tendency to lean forward too much, putting excessive strain on the lower back. But if you can master a ski machine, it is an excellent way to get fit. Stretching is vital to ski machine users because this exercise uses so many muscle groups.

AEROBICS CLASSES, STEP CLASSES, AND STAIR CLIMBERS

I've grouped these three modes of exercise together because they are surrounded by more misinformation than other forms of exercise.

Aerobics Classes

This is my favorite section of the entire book. What I am about to tell you is shocking, but it's all true.

I interviewed over a thousand women for this section and asked them, "How many women, including yourself, do you know who have ever vastly improved their body by taking aerobics classes?" All of them said zero, not one!

TIP 56

Even if you took eight aerobics classes a day, your body would never change to your desired level of satisfaction.

All one thousand women also believed that if they worked up a sweat, that meant they were burning calories; if they were burning calories, then they had to be losing weight; if they were losing weight, then they had to be getting thinner. Not only were they not getting thinner, but about half actually noticed that their bodies had *increased* in size.

Out of the thousand women, who ranged in age from seventeen to seventy-two, not one could jump rope for five minutes at 140 rpm without having to stop a number of times to catch her breath. Yet they were used to taking an hour to an hour and a half of aerobics classes, two to four times a week. Not only were the aerobics classes not changing their bodies, they were doing nothing to increase the women's fitness levels. How come aerobics classes are not an effective way to change your body as well as to get fit? Many reasons.

Remember the four phases of each workout? Do you also remember that I said you cannot get fit unless you complete each workout in that exact order? Moving your arms and legs around for a couple of minutes does not suffice as an effective warm-up. In most aerobics, exercise, or step classes the warm-up stage and stretch phase are combined as one.

TIP 57

Another problem with most exercise classes is that 60 to 70 percent of all participants injure themselves, and about half of those injuries are aches and pains that people will feel for the rest of their lives. Most injuries occur because of not properly warming up and stretching before going into the routines.

Another reason for the ineffectiveness of aerobics, step, and exercise classes is that most of the women who take them do not know how to perform each step or move correctly. Their body alignment is off, as is their balance. Very few exercisers can follow an instructor perfectly and also perform the exercise in a way that they are not injuring themselves.

Why then do people keep taking these classes? They take them because they believe that they are going to change their bodies. They take them because someone next to them appears to be fit and has a nice figure, and they think that they too will look like that if they participate in the same class. What they don't realize is that the person with the nice figure did not get that figure by taking exercise classes alone. She either achieved that good look through other fitness means or was blessed with a good body to start with. The class is just maintaining whatever fitness level she already has.

You *cannot* make positive changes to your problem areas through aerobics, step, or exercise classes. You can, however, make small improvements, such as lose weight, tone your upper and lower body, and increase abdominal strength slightly, if you follow the four phases in doing each workout and use perfect form with each movement.

Take aerobics classes on the days between your regular fitness regimen. Take them for fun, take them because you enjoy exercising with others. Take them because you want to improve your coordination.

TIP 58

Do not take any aerobics class with the expectation that you're actually going to get fit or change your body to your desired level of satisfaction—because you won't.

Step Classes and Stair Climbers

TIP 59

For certain body types, step classes and stair climbers can actually *increase* the size of your buttocks, thighs, and hips.

If you have a tendency to add bulk or size to your lower body, then participating in these exercises will only make your body bigger. Although step classes and stair climbers will give you a rounder rear end and firm up your legs, this will push the fat deposits on the outside of your legs and hips farther and farther outward.

All the traditional ways to exercise get you fit with what I call "inner-outer" fitness—meaning they build new muscle underneath (inner) and push fat deposits out (outer). Doing step classes and stair climbing will get you firm underneath your fat but will do nothing to firm up the outer part of your skin. The more you do these types of exercises, the worse it will become. Doing any type of exercise with heavy weights will also push these fat deposits farther out, as will doing squats and leg presses with weights.

TIP 60

Beware of riding a stationary bike with any sort of tension. The more tension or resistance you ride with, the bigger your legs will get.

Performing exercises with leg weights is also a no-no, as they to will add bulk to your lower body. Running up stairs or hills will do the same. The more weights you do with low reps, the bigger your body will get. If you wish to lose mass, especially in your lower body, this can only be achieved by combining very high repetitions with no weights. If you ride a stationary bike, light tension or resistance combined with high rpm (80–120) will help elongate your muscles and firm you up without building size.

TIP 61

Contrary to popular belief, you cannot convert fat into muscle. Fat and muscle are made up of different substances.

In order to lose mass, bulk, and size on your body you must first burn the fat through proper exercise, then build new muscle. All aerobic-type exercises will help take that mass away if they are the correct exercises for your body type. To firm your body, anaerobic-type exercises are the solution. However, there is one exercise that happens to do both—one exercise that enables you to lose weight, lose mass, and firm at the same time. This exercise can be done at any age and is good for any body type. That exercise is rope jumping.

TIP 62

A jump rope is the best fitness investment you can make.

First let's clear up some misconceptions about our little friend the jump rope. Contrary to popular opinion, rope jumping is relatively easy on your knees. Rope jumping has $1/7$ to $1/2$ the impact of running. You do not need a lot of ceiling height. The rope comes only about ten inches over your head when jumping.

Rope jumping is not a high-impact exercise, it is a low-impact exercise. When it is done properly, your feet should not leave the ground more than an inch. Unlike running, in which you land on your heels and all the stress goes to your back and knees, with rope jumping you land on the balls (front) of your feet, so that the stress is more equally distributed, putting more stress on your quadriceps (the front of your legs).

What sets rope jumping apart from any other exercise is that it develops so many areas of fitness. I have been jumping rope since I was ten and still haven't outgrown it. To me that's the most amazing thing about rope jumping; you never get bored, you can do it for the rest of your life and still physically challenge yourself along the way. Its benefits are numerous: it improves cardiovascular conditioning, strengthens and tones all major muscle groups, and is effective in fighting osteoporosis; it improves coordination, balance, agility, and timing because the arms must work in perfect unison with the legs; and it is excellent for weight loss or control (in fact you burn more fat with rope jumping than with any other exercise).

You can burn from 600 to 1,000 calories per hour when jumping (120–140 jumps per minute). Rope jumping is inexpensive, not dependent on weather, and can be performed practically anywhere.

The best jump ropes are those that are plastic or vinyl. These are easier to jump with than a cloth, nylon, or leather rope. To determine the correct length of a rope, stand with one foot on the middle of the rope. The ends of the rope handles should reach and barely touch right under the armpits. Quality cross-training shoes should be worn at all times because they provide lateral support and have cushioning under the forefoot to absorb the impact from jumping. Do not wear tennis or running shoes; they lend no support, and the soles may snag the rope while jumping.

TIP 63

The best surface to jump rope on is a "suspended" wooden floor, since it is stable yet dissipates the energy of impact by flexing a small amount.

Any wood surface is usually good, because wood has a natural give to it, unless the wood is laid over cement. Do not jump on a rug, because your feet tend to sink into the nap, which will also throw off your timing.

Start slowly and pay special attention to stretching your calves. Begin with two to four sets of 100 to 200 jumps per set. Try to average at least 100 revolutions per minute and build your pulse rate up to 150 beats per minute. The best thing about rope jumping is the "high" that it gives you. I have yet to find any exercise or combination of exercises that gives me the satisfaction of rope jumping. Believe it or not, that simple jump rope has changed more people's fitness levels, created more confidence and changed more lives for the better than the fountain of youth!

TIP 64

The most effective way to get rid of the fat on the outside of your legs right below your hips is with the jump rope. Rope jumping also is a very effective way of eliminating cellulite from your body.

If you can jump rope for six minutes at a relatively high intensity (140 rpm), it can be equivalent to thirty minutes of jogging. Rope jumping will vastly increase your aerobic capacity for jogging, but jogging only slightly improves your aerobic capacity for jumping rope. Jumping rope can help strengthen weak legs, knees, and ankles. For some, it can even strengthen legs with knee and ankle problems.

TIP 65

You can lose more weight by rope jumping than any other exercise, and it is a complete body workout, for it also tones your upper body.

For those of you who are saying, "I've never jumped rope before," it is very easy to do and learn. Once you get the feel for it, you'll be able to increase your skill as your coordination improves. Once you see all the different movements and tricks that can be done, you will never want to put that rope away. The key to this is patience and determination; once you achieve that, you're on your way to a new and improved you.

MUSCLE STRENGTHENING AND ENDURANCE EXERCISES, INCLUDING WEIGHT LIFTING

There are a number of techniques for increasing your total body strength and endurance. Some are safer than others, as well as more effective and efficient. The key to choosing the technique that works best for you is knowing what factors to consider—your lifestyle, your orthopedic background, and your body type.

TIP 66

If you choose to lift weights, remember, it's only one small piece of the pie toward getting fit. You must still perform other exercises in order to complete that pie.

Muscular strength is the maximum force that can be generated by a particular muscle. Someone with a lot of strength is capable of lifting heavy objects. Strength is dependent on the human body's ability to gather available muscle fibers.

Muscular endurance is the ability of a muscle to

perform repetitive contractions against a less than maximal load. The ability to lift a weight many times before becoming fatigued is a good indicator of muscular endurance.

How much muscular strength and muscular endurance are needed in order for us to live a productive life? Some people need higher levels than others because of their occupational or recreational pursuits.

TIP 67

It is difficult to determine the absolute level of muscular strength and endurance needed to combat the diseases associated with inactivity.

One thing is certain, and that is: if you have a weak upper body, you're more apt to have stress affect the neck, shoulders, and back regions of the body. Typically, fitness programs focus on attaining cardiorespiratory fitness and keeping body fat percentages at an acceptable level. Recently, though, health professionals are recognizing the need for abdominal muscle strength and endurance to help prevent or relieve low back pain.

Measures of Strength

Isometric strength refers to constant length; the muscle does not shorten. Isometric strength varies with the angle of the joint and does not provide a measure of strength throughout a joint's normal range of motion.

Two examples include gripping a hand grip, and pressing both your palms together as hard as you can for a period of time.

Isokinetic strength is measured with a special machine that controls the speed at which you can move a joint through its range of motion. When a muscle contracts with as much force as possible to move a part of your body, sensors in the machine measure strength throughout the range of motion. An example would be to have one of your legs attached to a lever arm that controls how fast that limb moves. This strength is usually measured and used for physical rehabilitation and training facilities.

Isotonic strength is measured as the heaviest weight lifted through a normal range of motion. Weight lifting is an example. How much weight you can bench press with one repetition is a good measure of how strong you are.

Muscular endurance can be increased over time with the proper training program. Chin-ups, push-ups, dips, and pull-ups are good examples of muscular endurance.

TIP 68

If your goal is to firm, tone, or reduce, you want to concentrate on developing good muscle endurance.

High repetitions with a small amount of weight will help you achieve your goals. If you want to build pure strength with some bulk and are trying to add size to your body, it's best to exercise using a heavy amount of weight in combination with low repetitions.

To improve its strength, a muscle must lift a heavier weight than that to which it is accustomed. As your muscle gets used to that new heavier load, you must overload the muscle again if you are to keep increasing your strength. As your strength increases, so does the size of your muscles. That's why lifting heavy weights will not reduce your body size as easily as working to increase your muscle endurance. You can increase your muscle endurance without vastly increasing your muscle size. Generally, the effects of training are specific to exercises performed; however, there is some overlap in the areas of strength and endurance. You cannot completely isolate one from the other.

Developing Muscle Strength and Muscle Endurance with Weights

Repetitions, also known as reps, represent the number of times you perform an exercise. Sets represent the number of repetitions done before a rest. Therefore, doing three sets of ten reps means performing an exercise for ten repetitions three separate times, for a total of thirty reps. For optimal gains in muscular strength, you should do three sets of five to ten reps.

When you can lift the weight more than ten reps, increase the weight. This will increase the load against which the muscle must work.

TIP 69

For optimal gains in muscular endurance, do three to five sets of ten to fifty reps. Do not increase the amount of weight; rather increase the number of reps you perform.

When starting a weight-training program, to increase your muscular strength, you should lift a weight equal to 1/4 to 1/3 of your body weight or less for upper body exercises, and a weight equal to 1/2 to 2/3 of your body weight or less for lower body exercises. Gradually add more weight as you feel more comfortable and confident that you can sustain it without hurting yourself.

Developing Muscle Strength and Muscle Endurance Without Weights

If you presently exercise by running, cycling, or jumping rope, you're probably maintaining an adequate level of muscular strength and endurance for your lower body. But these exercises might not be enough to help strengthen your arms, shoulders, stomach, and back.

One of the safest and most effective ways to increase muscle strength and endurance for your upper body is to work against your own body weight as resistance. Push-ups on your toes (or on your knees for those who are not strong enough) are a great exercise for developing arms, back, and shoulders. Pull-ups and chin-ups are also very effective but are very difficult. Most people cannot do one pull-up or chin-up.

Chins and pulls also help your abdominal and back muscles, and increase your range of motion. This fosters greater flexibility, strength, and endurance. Depending upon your age, men should be able to perform twenty-five to fifty push-ups and five to ten chins or pulls. Women should be able to do seven to fifteen push-ups and two to seven chins or pulls.

Another great exercise for developing muscular strength and endurance for your entire upper body are dips, and chair dips for those who are not strong enough.

TIP 70

Chair dips and regular dips provide the best exercise for firming the back of your arms (triceps).

In chapter 10 I will cover certain weight lifting exercises and techniques using a ten-pound curl bar or a fifteen-pound straight bar. If you exercise properly with either of these bars, it is more effective than using a roomful of machines and weights.

I'm not a big believer in lifting weights for fitness. First off, it can be dangerous. Second, it is *not* the best or fastest way to develop strength and endurance. Remember, almost all of us need endurance rather than strength, unless we are training for a particular sport that uses more strength than endurance, such as competitive bodybuilding. For most people (about 99 percent of us), muscle endurance is more relative to your daily activities and leisure sports.

TIP 71

An example of good muscular endurance: To have the ability to hit your tennis serve with the same velocity in game one as you do in game twenty-one, two hours later. Or, to be able to hit a golf ball 250 yards on the first hole and 250 yards on the eighteenth hole, four hours later.

Weights are too complicated: they require a spotter for a number of exercises, they are very time consuming, you cannot take them with you while traveling, they give you an artificial pumped-up look, you lose flexibility, and if lifted incorrectly they put a lot of undue stress on your joints and back. When you stop, your body loses tone and strength faster than with other means of exercise.

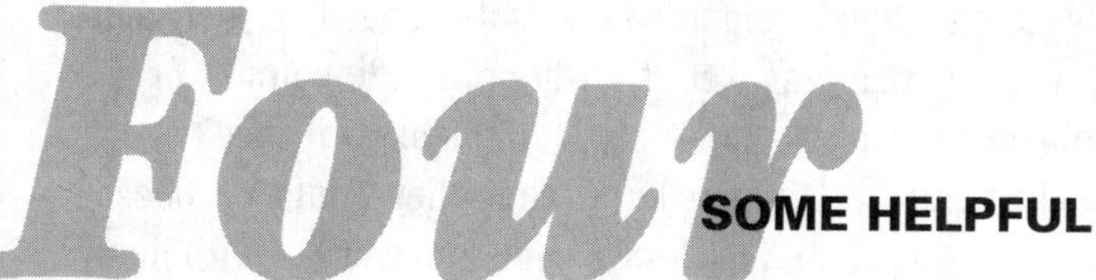

Four

SOME HELPFUL FACTS ABOUT YOUR BODY AND FITNESS

FAT COUNT FALLACY (WEIGHT LOSS VS. FAT LOSS)

So, you want to be thin, huh? How often do we stare with envy at some woman who stands about five feet eight and weighs in dripping wet at a whopping 120 pounds, or the models flashing across the runway who look as if they haven't eaten in months? Did you know that they could be obese? That's right, obese. In fact I have seen and worked with many obese women who do not even weigh 130 pounds. How is this possible?

TIP 72

Everyone's body composition is made up of lean body mass and body fat.

Lean body mass consists of the muscles, bones, nervous tissue, skin, and organs. Lean body mass represents the metabolically active part of our bodies that makes a positive contribution to energy production during exercise. Body fat represents body tissue that stores energy for use during some forms of exercise but otherwise does not directly aid exercise performance.

For men, 3 percent to 6 percent of your total body weight must be fat, the minimum necessary for maintenance of life and reproduction. For women, it is essential to have 8 percent to 12 percent.

TIP 73

For women, having an amount of body fat greater than or equal to 30 percent of your total body weight is considered obese. Your ideal level of body fat should be between 15 percent and 22 percent.

Body fat levels do change with age; however, an ideal percentage can be maintained at a good level throughout life with the proper exercise and diet.

As you can now see, many women who are five feet eight and weigh 120 pounds can easily be considered obese if 30 percent of their 120 pounds is fat. That means that out of her 120 pounds, 36 pounds are pure fat and the remaining 84 pounds are lean body mass. If that same woman possessed only 15 percent body fat, her numbers would look like this: 18 pounds of fat and 102 pounds of lean body mass.

The bigger boned you are and the more natural lean muscle you possess, the more body fat you can—and need to—carry. The smaller boned you are, and if you do not possess a lot of natural lean muscle, the less body fat you need.

T I P 7 4

Ideally, men should have between 10 percent and 15 percent body fat; a level equal to or greater than 23 percent is considered obese.

It is possible to be overweight but underfat. A man who stands six feet could weigh 220 pounds yet his body fat could be only 12 percent. That means that out of that 220 pounds, only 26 pounds is fat and the remaining 194 pounds is lean body mass.

According to most insurance company weight standards for men and women, a man of six feet with a large frame should weigh no more than 189 pounds. A good example of these overweight but underfat types are professional football players, especially the linebackers and running backs. They look huge, but their body fat is relatively low.

On the other side of the coin, you could be underweight but overly fat. Let's take a large-framed six-foot man who weighs 185 pounds with a body fat percentage of 25 percent. That represents over 46 pounds of fat and only 139 pounds of lean body mass. Even though the first man outweighs him by 35 pounds, he has 20 pounds less fat on him.

A good example of the type of person who is built like this is a typical overworked businessman. This person has a poor diet, sits a lot, suffers excessive stress, and exercises inconsistently.

Is it better to be overweight and underfat or underweight and overfat? The former is much better for you, because not only will you look and feel better, but you'd have to be a somewhat fit person to be overweight and underfat. If you're underweight and overfat, you are not only unfit but will appear to be heavier than you actually are.

There are a few ways to analyze body composition. A highly accurate version is underwater weighing, also known as hydrostatic weighing. This method measures body density by calculating the tendency of a person to sink when placed in water. Your weight is measured on land with a calibrated scale and again when you are completely submerged underwater. Body fat tends to float, so a lean person will weigh more underwater than a fat person. This technique is very accurate but time-consuming and expensive.

Another common way to determine your lean body mass vs. body fat is the skinfold caliper measurement. This technique is more commonly used and is done by measuring the thickness of several skinfolds. This technique is based on the theory that a large amount of the total body fat is located just under the skin, and by measuring an estimate of that fat, overall body fat can be determined. The skinfold measurement has about a 3 percent degree of error. Any local fitness club can measure your body fat with this technique.

TIP 75

The scale alone does not determine whether or not you've increased your lean body mass and reduced body fat. In fact, you could lose ten pounds by dieting and have actually gained body fat!

If you lose five pounds through proper exercise, you will look as if you lost ten pounds. You would have to lose ten pounds or more through dieting alone to get the same visual effect. And by the way, that visual effect is with your clothes on, not off. Naked, you might still look just as bad or worse if you lost the weight through dieting alone.

A simple technique to lose weight and decrease body fat works like this: Let's say that you take in 10 calories a day for seven days, which represents 70 calories taken in during a week. Let's also assume that you expend 10 calories a day, or 70 calories a week, through your normal work and play. You have tried every diet in existence, but none has worked. So now you increase your activity level during the week through proper exercise, but you do not alter your eating in any way. Now you're expending 20 calories a day yet consuming only 10 calories. You can easily see that by the end of the week, you will lose not only weight but body fat as well. Calories in must equal calories out.

The only thing you need to know about losing and keeping weight off for the rest of your life is:

TIP 76

Only through proper exercise will you be able to lose body fat and weight. Dieting alone will never get you to meet your weight, body fat percentage, and aesthetic goals.

I tell my clients to throw their scales away and use their mirror and clothes as their feedback. One week you could lose a lot of body fat but no weight, so what are you going to do, stop exercising in discouragement?

TIP 77

Most of you who are trying to lose weight should know that if you're losing more than three pounds a week, chances are you will not keep it off.

Women are especially impatient when it comes to losing weight. Right before the summer, I always get the same requests. "Edward, I want to lose ten pounds in two weeks." I respond, "You did not gain those ten pounds in two weeks, why do you think you'll lose them in two weeks?" "But Edward, I've lost it *before*," they reply. I say, "That's right, you have lost it before, but it has not stayed off because you lost it too fast, and your body could not take the stress and shock you put it through."

I don't care how much willpower a person has; when the body says, "feed me," the mind will always yield, unless artificially assisted by drugs or other means.

Read further and see how much ten pounds of weight loss in five weeks represents. If you weigh 130 pounds, a surefire game plan is to lose two pounds a week for five weeks and keep it off for life by exercising on a regular basis. How would you like to weigh 140 pounds in five weeks instead of 130? You see how much two pounds a week truly represents? When you look at it like that, five weeks is not all that much time now, is it? Imagine how much weight and body fat you could lose over time if you changed your eating habits and decreased your caloric intake by just 10 percent.

HOW MUCH ENERGY DO YOU USE WHILE EXERCISING?

If you and I were sitting around watching television for a couple of hours and we each ate a candy bar, most likely you would gain more weight than me and that candy bar would add more body fat to your body than mine.

TIP 78

The more fit you are, the more calories you burn up while being sedentary.

Your metabolism is defined as the chemical and physical processes in the body that provide energy for the maintenance of life. There are a number of factors that determine your metabolism—genetics, diet, stress, sleep, activity level, fitness level, and certain medical conditions, among others. To raise your metabolism simply means that your body is working more efficiently.

Why do some individuals have more energy than others, and what exactly is energy? Energy is defined as the body's capacity to perform work. It is often measured in terms of oxygen consumption. Although we know the caloric value of certain foods, determining the caloric value (in terms of total calories burned) of exercise varies with the type of activity or exercise, the intensity level, and the weight of the individual performing the exercise.

TIP 79

Typically, the average person burns between 200 and 300 calories (cals) for every hour of exercise.

We can use this figure in determining and measuring the energy costs of exercise and activity. For every liter of oxygen used, the body uses 5 cals. In our resting state, when we are not moving about or exercising, we use up and burn about 1 cal per hour for every 2.2 pounds of body weight. The energy associated with sitting at rest is the largest energy-producing task for most Americans today!

If you rest during the entire day, you use 1 cal per hour for every 2.2 pounds of your total body weight. This is what is referred to as your basal metabolic rate (BMR).

TIP 80

To find your BMR in terms of how many calories you burn during rest throughout the course of the day, multiply 24 (hours) times your body weight divided by 2.2, or multiply 11 times your body weight in pounds. 1887.27

So, a 140-pound person uses about 1,540 calories a day at their resting rate. Now, add between 400 and 1,000 calories, depending how active you are, and that total number represents how many calories you will burn that day. That number also represents how many calories you should be consuming in order to maintain your weight. If you exceed that total, you'll gain weight; if you consume fewer calories, you will lose weight. It does not matter if you exceed that number of calories by eating lettuce, carrots, or pizza, you will still gain weight. Also keep in mind that if you reduce your caloric intake too much, your body responds by *decreasing* its resting metabolic rate in order to protect its limited energy stores. That's why a lot of people either stop losing weight when they crash-diet or may even gain weight.

Losing weight by dieting alone represents approximately a 50–60 percent loss of muscle and lean body mass.

The following are the best calorie-burning activities and exercises (figures are based on a 150-pound individual performing exercise for one hour).

750–900 cals./hour:
Rope jumping, squash, cross-country skiing, soccer, full-court basketball, handball, racquetball, boxing, backpacking, paddleball, and snowshoeing.

500–750 cals./hour:
Two-hand touch football, tennis, badminton, canoeing, rowing, kayaking, aerobic dancing, mountain climbing, cycling, hiking, horseback riding, hunting small game, scuba diving, roller blading, roller skating, ice skating, water skiing, downhill skiing, sledding and tobogganing, swimming, judo, karate, jogging, fast walking, fencing, and field hockey.

200–500 cals./hour:
Golf, walking at a slow pace, archery, bowling, social dancing, horseshoe pitching, sailing, shuffleboard, table tennis, and volleyball.

Depending upon your intensity level (energy exerted) and weight, you can burn up to another 200 to 400 calories an hour for some of these activities and exercises. For instance, if you play golf and walk the course—or better yet, walk while pulling or carrying clubs—you will burn up a heck of a lot more calories than by riding in a cart.

TIP 82

Don't be obsessed with counting how many calories you are actually burning during exercise. It is very difficult to accurately determine an exact number.

It really does not matter how many calories you are burning so long as you exercise regularly and increase the intensity over time. What's more important is the type of exercise you choose. If you are trying to lose weight, then choose an exercise that has a tendency to burn more calories, even if you start slowly with that particular exercise. With time, you will increase your intensity level.

Now you can plainly see that merely walking on a treadmill for forty-five minutes a day does not guarantee weight loss. More important, utilizing a treadmill alone will never get you fit!

EXERCISE AND YOUR TARGET HEART RATE ZONE

One reason that many people exercising each day are not increasing their fitness level and reaching their weight loss goals is that they're not exercising in their target heart rate zone. There is a lot of controversy over what each individual's *zone* should be during exercise.

TIP 83

As your age increases, the recommended number of heartbeats per minute during exercise decreases because of the strain you put on your heart.

Your target heart rate (THR) is defined as the heart rate recommended for exercising. When you're in your target heart rate zone, it means you're exercising just vigorously enough. Exercising above your THR means you're out of your zone (exercising too vigorously), and exercising below your THR is referred to as under your zone (not exercising vigorously enough).

How hard should you work during exercise? The amount of energy (intensity) of exercise is the overload you place on your cardiorespiratory system during a workout. The threshold needed to achieve benefits is lower for those who are very sedentary compared to the very fit. Other factors such as age, primary risk factors (smoking, heart disease, high blood pressure) and secondary risk factors (over forty-five years of age, family history of heart disease, very stressful lifestyle, among others) dictate how hard one should work while starting or maintaining an exercise program. (See the section on cardiovascular risk factors at the end of this chapter.)

TIP 84

How your heart will react when you begin an exercise program or add new exercises to your current routine has a lot to do with how active and fit you *presently* are.

Estimating Cardiac Risk

Here's an example: Who do you think is more at risk for a heart attack, Bob or Peter? Bob does nothing but work every day in a highly stressful environment, is married with two children, and plays golf and tennis about twice a month. He lives in New York City and is forty-eight years old; he is six feet, about 180 pounds, medium frame; he does not smoke, drinks only on weekends, has no family history of heart disease, and got a clean bill of health at his last physical.

Peter is forty-five years old, six feet, large framed, weighs about 220 pounds and is twenty pounds overweight. In addition, he smokes around ten cigarettes a day and drinks two to four times a week, but never more than two or three drinks of hard alcohol. Peter's father, who died of a heart attack at fifty-four years of age, never exercised. Peter travels with his work about twice a month. He, too, is a family man and has three children. Peter is very active, plays golf or tennis on weekends, and also swims every weekend in sunny southern California. In addition, Peter works out three times a week like clockwork. No matter what, Peter bikes, lifts weights, runs, and jumps rope for an hour each time he exercises.

Now, on paper, Bob appears less at risk for having a heart attack. But the hidden factor here is that Bob's heart is never challenged. How hard should he work if he were to engage in exercise? Peter's heart, on the other hand, is used to his jumping up and down, especially since he combines aerobic exercise and anaerobic exercise. If Bob and Peter were to run a mile, which one would you bet on to cross the finish line first? Bob might not even cross the finish line, but I'll bet you dollars to doughnuts that Peter blows him away!

Determining Your Heart Rate Zone

People have a tendency to begin an exercise program either under or over their zone. And very few warm up or stretch prior to increasing the intensity (energy) level. Remember, your heart rate increases faster when you're performing anaerobic as opposed to aerobic exercise.

TIP 85

A good way to judge how hard you should be exercising is to see how high your heart rate is during the activity, since heart rate

increases when intensity (energy) increases.

To determine your maximal heart rate zone, follow these steps: First you need to estimate what your maximal heart rate should be while exercising. Take the number 220 and subtract your age in years. This number represents your age-adjusted maximal heart rate. *Example:* for a sixty-year-old person, 220 – 60 = 160.

This number means that during *any* type of physical activity or exercise, your heart rate should not exceed 160 beats per minute. There are exceptions to this, for a well-trained athlete or certain professional athletes who have worked up to this level of (energy) intensity, for instance. But for most of you, you should monitor your heart rate during your exercise period in order to prevent overexerting yourself.

Now that you have your maximal heart rate, the second step toward determining your zone is to calculate 70 percent of your maximal heart rate, which is considered the *low* end of your zone when exercising. *Example:* 160 x .70 = 112. That means that in order to gain some benefit from exercise, you must work hard enough during the exercise for your heart to beat at least 112 beats per minute.

Next, calculate 85 percent of your maximal heart rate to determine the *high* end of your zone. *Example:* 160 x .85 = 136. So, a sixty-year-old individual should be exercising just hard enough for the heart to beat between 112 and 136 beats per minute. Now you know what is meant by exercising in your target heart rate zone.

TIP 86

When beginning an exercise program, make sure you're exercising so that your heart rate is toward the low end of your heart rate zone.

I strongly recommend that anyone over thirty-five years of age get a stress test done (EKG, ECG) prior to engaging in *any* exercise or activity that causes their heart rate to go from its standing pulse to 70 percent of their maximal heart rate. This, by the way, includes most activities.

TIP 87

When starting out, it's more important to increase your time (period) than increasing intensity (energy). Also, participate in low-intensity exercises, such as riding a stationary bike or walking on a treadmill.

If you're completely sedentary, you can ride a stationary bike at a moderate speed (60 rpm) with low to moderate tension for fifteen minutes or more; then you can increase the workload. Increasing the tension on the bike will raise your heart rate faster than increasing the time pedaling at the same rpm.

Remember to monitor your progress. To monitor your heart rate during exercise all you need to do is find your pulse on various parts of your body. You can also purchase a heart rate monitor, which gives you your heart rate while exercising (a good device will cost between $75 to $150) but these are not always reliable because of the jarring your body creates performing the exercise. I do, however, recommend that people with any heart complications use one. You can easily see if you are out of your zone and immediately lower your intensity (energy).

To monitor your heart rate manually, stop exercising and within five seconds count the pulse at your neck, wrist, temple, or chest for ten seconds. Your heart rate drops very quickly when you stop exercising, so it's imperative to gauge the number of beats within five seconds in order to get an accurate reading.

Place the tips of the index and middle fingers (not the thumb, which has a pulse of its own) over the artery and press lightly when taking your pulse from your neck, wrist, or temple. When taking your pulse on your chest, place the heel of your right hand over the left side of your chest. At the same time, look at a second hand on a clock or watch and count the number of times you feel a pulse, for ten seconds.

When you have the number of beats for ten seconds, multiply that number times six (six times your number of pulse beats for ten seconds). That number represents how many times your heart is beating per minute during exercise. That number should be in your zone. If not, adjust your intensity (energy) level.

Take your pulse a number of times during exercise if you feel that you're either above or under your zone. With practice you won't even have to check your pulse; you'll know how hard you're working. Another way to determine if you're overdoing it during your workout is recognizing a shortness of breath, not being able to talk comfortably, dizziness, or a feeling of nausea. If you experience any of these symptoms, you should stop exercising immediately and place a wet, cool towel on your head and lie down on your back with your feet level with your head.

TIP 88

If you're just starting to exercise, remember that the more risk factors you have, the more critical it is for you to exercise closer to the low end or even under the low end of your zone.

Your zone is only a range and guide to follow. If you are exercising and find you're huffing and puffing, check your pulse. If you are still under your zone, decrease the intensity (energy) level immediately. Even though you're under your prescribed zone, you are still getting benefits from the exercise. With time, you will be able to exercise comfortably within your zone, and you'll even have to increase it. Don't get discouraged.

Just remaining in your zone during your workout doesn't necessarily mean you are becoming more fit or that your body will change in the areas that you expect it to. You could be doing the wrong type of exercise for your body type. For example, if you have a spoon-shaped body and are using step classes as your primary means of exercise, you'll never change your body to your desired level of satisfaction. Sure, you'll become a little more fit, but if you can become more fit *and* change your body to your desired level of satisfaction at the same time, why wouldn't you?

TIP 89

Everyone's system and body react differently to exercise. No two bodies are exactly alike.

If your body is not responding positively to the type of exercises that you're currently performing, or you need help in engaging in a proper and regular fitness program, please inquire about our FastFitness routine. We will design an exercise regimen specifically for your body type as well as your orthopedic and medical background. Contact:

Exude Inc.
16 East 52nd Street
3rd Floor
New York, NY 10022
1–800–24-EXUDE or (212) 644-9559
Fax: (212) 759-4387
Web site: exude.com

CARDIOVASCULAR RISK FACTORS

The American Heart Association and American College of Sports Medicine list primary and secondary risk factors for coronary heart disease as follows:

PRIMARY

1. Major alterable risk factors: These are factors that can be modified.

   A. Physical inactivity
   B. Smoking—#l preventable health problem
   C. High blood pressure (140/90)
   D. High cholesterol levels
      1. desirable: below 200 mg/dl
      2. moderate risk: 200–239 mg/dl
      3. high risk: 240 mg/dl

2. Major unalterable risk factors: These are factors that can't be modified. Persons in these groups have a greater risk of heart disease, particularly if they adopt unhealthy behaviors.

   A. Those with a family history of heart disease
   B. Increasing age: men over 40, women over 50
   C. Men
   D. African Americans

SECONDARY

The following secondary risk factors contribute to increasing an individual's risk of CHD:

A. Obesity
B. High-fat diet
C. Stress

D. Extreme Type A personality
E. Diabetes

IDENTIFY YOUR RISK FACTORS

Primary risk factors

1. Sedentary lifestyle
2. Smoking
3. Family history of coronary heart disease (CHD) prior to age 50
4. Blood pressure over 140/90
5. Measured cholesterol level over 240
6. Abnormal ECG, chest and/or heart pain

Secondary risk factors

1. Age: Men 40+, Women 50+
2. Sex: male
3. Family history of CHD prior to age 60
4. Obesity—over 30% body fat
5. Extremely stressful lifestyle
6. Diabetes

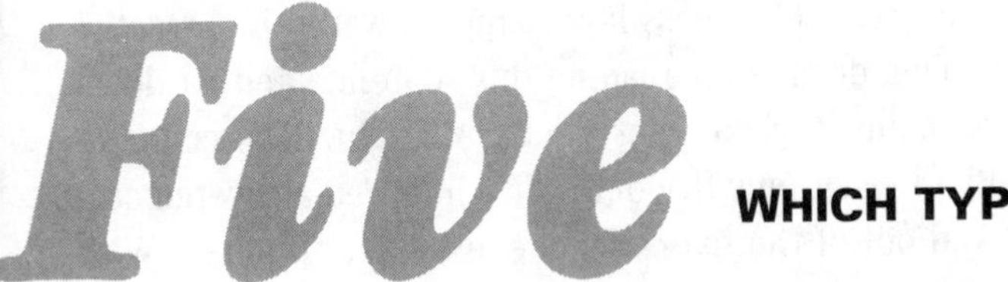

WHICH TYPE OF EXERCISE IS BEST SUITED FOR YOU?

A LESSON ON AEROBIC EXERCISE

I asked five hundred people the following question: "What is aerobic exercise?" Guess how many answered it correctly! Put this book down after reading this sentence and jot down what you think aerobic exercise is. All right, let's compare notes. By the way, only five out of five hundred answered correctly. And out of the five, only one answered in detail. With all that is written, seen, and heard on exercise, that's not a high percentage, is it?

Well, if most people cannot even comprehend or understand a simple term such as *aerobic exercise,* I guess exercise isn't that simple, is it? What I don't understand is how an educated person who spends ten years doing the same work, like practicing medicine, or accounting, can possibly think they know how to work out properly after watching a buddy, reading a single fitness article, or by watching a celebrity on television selling the latest exercise fad.

TIP 90

Aerobic exercise is defined as: sustained, rhythmic large-muscle activity that does not require more than a low or moderate intensity (energy) level and can be performed continuously without undue respiratory discomfort.

Some examples of aerobic exercise are: walking, jogging, rope jumping, swimming, cycling, cross-country skiing, and aerobics. *Aerobics* does not mean aerobic exercise, but it is a form of aerobic exercise just as the above-mentioned are.

TIP 91

It is commonly believed that in order to gain aerobic benefits from exercise, one must perform that aerobic-type exercise for twenty minutes or more. This is not so.

If you can walk or run only ten city blocks (approximately one-half mile), and it takes you only ten minutes to do so, did you improve your aerobic capacity? You bet your life you did! But if you are used to walking or running much more than that, then you probably did not improve your aerobic capacity.

To prove this point even further, if you walk or jog that half mile every day, and after two weeks you are capable of walking or jogging one mile, did you increase your aerobic capacity when you were only walking or jogging that half mile in ten minutes? Of course! Otherwise, you never would have been able to walk or jog the one mile. Did it take twenty minutes to walk or jog that half mile? No.

TIP 92

You can gain aerobic benefits and increase your aerobic capacity by exercising for only a couple of minutes or less.

Rope jumping is a good way of gaining aerobic benefits, yet you may be able to perform the exercise for only two minutes when starting out. In fact, for many who start working out with a jump rope, it could actually be anaerobic, and as you get in better cardiovascular condition, the rope jumping will become aerobic for you. You can also greatly increase your aerobic capacity by performing anaerobic exercises such as weight lifting, if you lift the weights for endurance instead of strength.

How important is aerobic exercise, and how does it benefit us? Aerobic fitness is a good measure of your heart's ability to pump oxygen-rich blood to your major muscles. (The following words are often used in conjunction with aerobic fitness: *cardiovascular and cardiorespiratory fitness.*) The healthier your heart is, the larger your heart becomes, which enables your body to pump greater volumes of blood with each beat more efficiently than with an unhealthy heart. This represents the most important benefit of exercise and is the primary physiological reason to improve your aerobic capacity.

If you want to get bigger and stronger, spend less time pumping weights and devote a little more time to cycling, running, or rope jumping. You'll meet your aesthetic goals quicker.

During aerobic exercise, your heart rate rises slowly to a point (hopefully within your zone) and stays at a certain level for a prolonged period. Although your heart rate will go up and down, it will rise or fall only slowly and in small increments. That is why you can perform aerobic-type exercises such as marathon running over an extended period of time. Aerobic exercise means exercise that requires the presence of oxygen. You must have a constant supply of oxygen delivered to the working muscles by circulating blood in order to sustain the exercise.

Risk during aerobic exercise is considerably less than with anaerobic exercise. It's during anaerobic exercise that your heart rate rises very quickly and fluctuates up and down, creating much more of a shock to your system and strain on your heart.

There are a number of ways to analyze your cardiorespiratory fitness level. If you have no major medical problems, you can participate in the following types of tests, but I would recommend getting your doctor's okay before engaging in *any* type of exercise, especially if you're over thirty-five and/or have medical problems.

A submaximal fitness test does not require you to exercise at your maximum effort, and it reduces the chance that you'll have sore muscles the next day. Heart rate and blood pressure are usually measured, and the test ends when you have reached between 70 percent and 85 percent of your estimated maximal heart rate.

If the measurements are normal, you can start an exercise program; if not, you should get additional tests. With some individuals, the submaximal test is continued and they are exercised to maximum. Conversely in some submaximal tests, no measurements are made other than the time it takes to run a specific distance (not recommended for sedentary people).

During the submaximal test you can walk on a treadmill, step up and down on a bench, or ride a stationary bike through a series of progressively more difficult stages until you reach a predetermined end point. Then when you reach 70 to 85 percent of your estimated maximal heart rate, the test ends. You are then judged on what is called Borg's Rating of Perceived Exertion (RPE). In this scale (0–10), higher scores reflect a more intense perception of effort; for example, the expression "very, very hard" (10) indicates near-maximal work.

Repeating the submaximal test after a few weeks is a good way to gauge progress and increased aerobic capacity in those who are exercising on a regular basis. One of the best ways to judge if you're in better cardiovascular condition is by looking at your heart rate (measured in beats per minute) performing the same exercise, at the same workload, for the same period of time. So, if your heart rate after fifteen minutes of walking at 4 mph was 120 beats per minute one month ago, and today it was 110 beats per minute, you have increased your aerobic capacity. Your heart rate will be slower at any given stage of the test as your cardiovascular level improves.

I'm not a big believer in testing sedentary people to their max or even 85 percent of their max. Too many things can go wrong. I recommend that those beginning a fitness program purchase a stationary bike and start out cycling at between 40 and 60 rpm, with very little tension or resistance. Ride for five minutes and take your pulse. Then adjust if you need to, noting how you feel and how close you are to your heart rate zone. Increase the time (period) by two to five minutes per week and the speed to 60 or 80 rpm, working up to a half hour. When you can cycle for a half hour at between 60 and 80 rpm, then start to increase the tension or resistance slightly. This increase in your workload will challenge your aerobic capacity.

Performing push-ups is not aerobic; you're using smaller muscle groups (i.e. arms and shoulders), which is why you can perform push-ups for only a short time. In addition, doing push-ups raises your heart rate very quickly, and it does not stabilize at a level low enough or long enough for you to take in sufficient oxygen to sustain the exercise. Conversely, jogging utilizes large muscle groups (i.e. legs) and can be sustained for a longer period of time because your heart rate does not rise as quickly and stays relatively steady during the duration of exercising, allowing you to take in more oxygen.

What truly distinguishes aerobic from anaerobic exercise is your heart rate while performing an exercise. Aerobic exercise cannot be performed at 85 to 100 percent of your estimated maximal heart rate for long periods of time. Lean toward a type of exercise that you like. If you do not like to jog, don't go out and buy a treadmill because your best pal has been bragging about how he loves his. Rule with your head when it comes to improving your heart.

EXERCISING ANAEROBICALLY

"Exercising without the presence of oxygen" is the scientific definition of *anaerobic.* How can you possibly exercise without oxygen? The term "without oxygen" refers to your body's inability to take in as much oxygen as it needs during aerobic exercise. This is because during anaerobic exercise your heart rate zooms upward, preventing your body from taking in oxygen as readily.

Examples of anaerobic exercise include: weight lifting; sit-ups, pull-ups, and chin-ups; push-ups, stomach crunches, and leg curls; using weight machines; running up a flight of stairs; running a 100-yard dash; shoveling snow; mowing the lawn; water and downhill skiing; ice skate sprinting; and all racquet sports. What do all these activities have in common? They are all stop-and-go in nature and require short bursts of energy to perform.

Exercising with breaks is also a good way to understand anaerobic exercise. Your body requires a break because your heart rate is closer to maximum than during aerobic exercise, when it beats at a lower rate and does not require you to stop to get your breath.

Some exercises and sports are a combination of both aerobic and anaerobic (i.e., full-court basketball, hockey).

TIP 94

Certain exercises traditionally labeled aerobic "act" anaerobically during the first five minutes or so.

For instance, many people who use a stair climber for their aerobic exercise find themselves out of breath after just two to four minutes on the stepper. Scientific and medical books, and fitness experts, agree that stair climbers provide a form of anaerobic exercise, because for the first couple of minutes, people who are using the stepper are toward the high end of their heart rate zone and may even be over it for a brief time. They might have to stop for a minute or so, catch their breath, and continue. Remember, aerobic = continuous = without a break. If you start rope jumping, which is also considered aerobic, and can jump rope for only one minute, rest, one minute, rest, and so on, don't you think you're getting aerobic benefits from the rope jumping? Of course you are. However, you are also gaining anaerobic benefits at the same time. You gain both aerobic and anaerobic benefits during the stop-and-go rope jumping, because during the one-minute segments of jumping, your heart rate rises very quickly toward the high end of your zone. Thus your heart gains the benefits of putting more demands upon it than if you were to work out at the low end of your zone. That is the reason why you have to stop after one minute of certain aerobic exercises. The same exercise performed at the same intensity and duration by two individuals can be aerobic for one and anaerobic for the other because of differing levels of cardiorespiratory fitness.

At Exude, we have found that one of the best methods for increasing one's aerobic capacity is to extend the period of time that one performs an anaerobic exercise. We have come up with different formulas that burn fat more efficiently with this methodology. Traditionally, it is believed that you burn more fat with aerobic exercise during long, sustained activity than with anaerobic exercises. This couldn't be farther from the truth. During anaerobic exercise, your heart rate is higher and your intensity (energy) is also higher. This means that you are actually burning more calories and fat during anaerobic exercise. However, it is difficult to sustain that type of exercise for a long period of time.

TIP 95

The better shape you're in, the less oxygen you use, because you possess a greater margin of reserve and are capable of continuing on a high performance level for a longer period of time without distress to your body.

Endurance-type exercises add to your cardiorespiratory reserves. Conversely, strength-type exercises do little to enhance your cardiovascular system. Both types of exercise are considered anaerobic. One great benefit of endurance-type exercises is that they protect your body from injury. The more fatigued you are, the more susceptible you are to injury. When you put physical demands on your body that it cannot sustain, something has to give. That's why so many individuals hurt themselves during downhill skiing. It's during that last run that their knee gives out.

TIP 96

If you injure yourself while exercising or playing a sport, listen to your body. The cardinal rule is: stop when your body says to stop. The pain will not go away if you continue, and in fact it most likely will get worse.

Exhaustion while exercising is anaerobically in the working muscles due to a buildup of lactic acid. If the removal of lactic acid by the circulatory system cannot keep pace with its accumulation, temporary muscular fatigue occurs with painful symptoms—this is the burn that you feel when doing your arm curls or stomach crunches. Most of you have read elsewhere and believe that you burn more fat through aerobic, not anaerobic, exercise. Not necessarily so. True, you do use more fatty acids as fuel during aerobic exercise. And with anaerobic exercise, you use more glucose (carbohydrates) as fuel. Only when you use up your glucose do you use your reserves, which would be your fatty acids with anaerobic exercise. Recently there has been much controversy about whether you can burn as much or more fat during anaerobic or aerobic exercise. But you can definitely lose weight and fat during anaerobic exercise, especially if you can train yourself to perform certain anaerobic-type exercises for prolonged periods of time.

TIP 97

Anaerobic-type exercises are best for allowing your body to become toned and firmed. Since so many different exercises overlap and give you both anaerobic and aerobic benefits, it's vital that you have a true understanding of how to perform these exercises with the correct form and body alignment.

Another example of combined anaerobic and aerobic exercise is walking or jogging with hand weights or wearing weights on another part of the body. Is there any benefit to bearing these weights? Yes, and no. Adding extra weights to your body during exercise increases the intensity (energy), which will raise your heart rate as well. If you do want to use weights during exercise, make sure you're orthopedically sound. Too many people who use hand weights and ankle weights put excess strain on their ankles, knees, lower back, and hips.

I do not recommend carrying or wearing weights for anyone, unless you enjoy hunting, backpacking, or other activities requiring weights to be incorporated into your training program. A lot of people develop severe medical problems because of adding weights to their bodies during exercise.

TIP 98

When starting an exercise program, perform more aerobic than anaerobic-type exercises. They're safer, and you can always add more anaerobic exercises as you get in better cardiovascular shape.

Remember that your heart rate is more likely to go out of your zone during anaerobic activity. And, as you do get more aerobically fit, you'll be able to put more physical demands upon your heart, preparing it for such anaerobic work.

LOSING WEIGHT VS. FIRMING AND TONING

TIP 99

If you're trying to lose weight through fitness, never allow more than one day to pass without aerobic exercise. It's better to exercise every day for forty-five

minutes than every two days for an hour and a half.

You need to keep burning up the calories that you consume each day. To lose weight, do not be too concerned with the scale initially. Remember, you can lose fat without losing pounds on the scale. I recommend weighing yourself once a month, in the morning, on the same day each month.

TIP 100

Because there are so many factors that can determine weight loss for any given week, define your goals with weight loss on a monthly basis.

If you have only ten to twenty pounds to lose, make your goal four pounds of weight loss a month. If you need to lose between twenty-one and forty pounds, make your goal six pounds of weight loss a month. If you need to lose more than forty pounds, make your goal eight pounds a month until you get down in weight, then adjust your goal to six pounds a month, and for the home stretch—four pounds a month.

TIP 101

In the beginning of a weight loss program, fitness is more

important than your diet total amount of calories y consume).

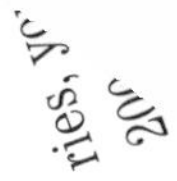

Even if you do not reduce your total amount consumed, with increased activity you will los Total calories taken in minus total calories use weight gain or weight loss. Review the formula in c 4 to figure out how many calories you need to maintain your weight during inactivity. As you begin to lose weight, and your body and mind have adjusted to regular exercise, then it's time to sit down with a nutritionist and review your diet.

TIP 102

Do not try to start an exercise program while trying to alter your diet drastically. If you do, chances are you'll fail at both.

Initially, exercise is more important than diet for losing weight. It has approximately five to ten times the overall impact. If you eat or drink too much on any given evening, the next day you can work it off with proper exercise. But if you try to work it off by dieting, it could take days or even weeks.

Let's take a look at some numbers: Saturday night you drink three glasses of wine and eat cheese, crackers, peanuts, a sensible dinner, and for dessert a piece of cheesecake. You have consumed approximately 1,200 extra calories that day. In order to lose that 1,200 calo-

.. would have to cut back on your food intake by . calories a day for six straight days. Now, it's awfully hard to be good for six straight days. Besides, who wants to? Learn to live your life in moderation.

That's what's great about fitness and exercise: if you have an off day, you can make it up through proper exercise. Life is short, so enjoy it to the hilt, but be in control.

TIP 103

If you are going to overeat, eat carbohydrates and proteins, because it's much more difficult for your body to transform these into body fat, whereas dietary fat quickly moves into your fat cells as if it has radar.

One of my theories on fat is as follows: when proteins and carbohydrates enter your body, they are dispersed more evenly throughout. For some strange and currently unknown reason, fat enters the body and goes right to an area or areas on the body where fat deposits build up and collect. These regions of fat buildup vary from person to person and are usually genetically determined.

(I do not include a separate section on nutrition in this book because, like exercise and fitness, it is an art. It would take another book in and of itself to fully understand nutrition and food intake. I do however make occasional references to emphasize or help you to better understand a particular point.)

If losing weight is your goal, purchase a tape measure and an accurate scale. Weigh yourself on the same scale every time you weigh in.

TIP 104

The biggest drawback of weighing yourself too often is the "highs and lows" you experience when you look at the number on the scale.

Measuring yourself around your problem areas is a better indication of whether your body is changing for the better. You could lose inches from your thighs and hips but only a couple of pounds at most. Measure yourself once a month. There will be times when you'll lose more one month than the next. Although the tape measure will not give you a precise reading on total weight loss or body fat loss through exercise, it is a sound reading of progress.

The scale comes into play when your goal is to lose weight and you find yourself losing inches, but not as much weight for the total inches that are evaporating from your body. This usually means that your diet needs to be altered. Start to keep a food and exercise log if this happens. Perhaps you are not increasing your period (time) enough, or your energy (intensity) enough. It could be you're still consuming too many calories even though you have cut out most of your fatty favorites.

Genetics and metabolism play an integral part in achieving your goals. They won't prevent you from achieving your goals, but they can influence the speed at which your goals will be met. Still, the most important factor for achieving weight loss with fitness is being consistent with proper exercise for your body type.

On the psychological side of the equation, I have found that those individuals who are presently overweight (I don't care if it is ten pounds or a hundred) but were once in shape or at least comfortable with the way they once looked, are very successful in achieving their weight loss goals. Those individuals whose perception is that they were never in shape or "thin" before, and have had a weight problem their entire life, have more difficulty in achieving weight loss goals.

TIP 105

With fitness, as in life, it's not where you are, it's where you're going.

I'm not a big believer in analyzing why someone is overweight. But I am a firm believer in analyzing your present circumstances, lifestyle, and perceived constraints in order to find a new recipe for a more effective and efficient way to live your life. Anyone can change how they look and feel if properly motivated and taught.

The happy and overweight person has to get fit *twice* in order to get fit at all. First, you have to start losing weight, which will allow your body to look and behave differently. Second, you have to be aware of the changes that are taking place. Ten pounds of weight loss on someone who has been very overweight their entire life might draw a yawn for some. Others would give their right arm to lose those same ten pounds. It's all a matter of perception.

AN EXPLANATION OF SOME "BEST" EXERCISES FOR WEIGHT LOSS

The following are the best exercises to perform if your goal is to lose weight. (All of chapter 10 is devoted to full-body workouts.) Assuming you are orthopedically sound and have clearance from your doctor, if you incorporate these types of exercises into your workout correctly, they will help lead to a leaner and trimmer body.

If you have only half an hour to devote to the aerobic component of our total workout, the number one exercise for losing weight is rope jumping, the number two exercise is cross-country skiing or simulation, number three is full-court basketball, and the next exercises are about equal: squash, handball, paddleball, racquetball, jogging (running), backpacking, hiking, soccer, aerobics, and cycling. If you're not orthopedically sound and have not received clearance from your doctor to perform any of these exercises, ask him or her about performing the next best exercise, which is riding a recumbent stationary bike at high rpm with moderate tension or resistance. Swimming and walking are some of the most time-consuming weight loss exercises you can perform, unless you are walking at a speed of at least 5.0 miles per hour. Most people who can walk at that speed for half an hour or more typically do not need to lose a heck of a lot of weight.

Don't forget to include the four phases of every workout (see chapter 2) each time you exercise. They'll help you achieve your weight-loss goals faster, and your chances for injuring yourself decrease vastly. Also, if you cannot perform any of the above exercises for at least half an hour, don't give up. With time and perseverance, you will eventually be able to go the whole route plus more. If you are physically capable of performing any of the above exercises and you find yourself having to stop frequently in the beginning to rest, do so; catch your breath and do some more.

Do not make substitutions for any of these exercises unless they are harming your body.

TIP 106

Don't substitute walking for rope jumping because it's easier to do. Work on disciplining yourself and pushing yourself within safe measures. The difference between rope jumping and walking for weight loss is about a ten-to-one ratio as far as time is concerned, not to mention all the other benefits rope jumping brings you that walking can *never* bring you.

TIP 107

You cannot vastly reduce the size of your stomach by doing sit-ups or any other stomach exercise. You can, however, *firm* your stomach by performing sit-ups and other stomach exercises.

The rule of thumb for firming and toning your body is simple: anaerobic-type exercises are the best for firming, and aerobic-type exercises are best for losing weight and taking away mass from your body. The key to getting fit *and* changing your body is determining how much aerobic or anaerobic exercise your fitness regimen should include. We're going to call this mixture your *formula*. This is similar to the REPS principle discussed in chapter 2 (recurrence, energy, period, and sort). But your formula describes the sort (type) of exercise you should do (according to your goals and body type) by prescribing the ratio of aerobic to anaerobic exercise.

There are a couple of things to consider when you are designing your formula. Given one hour of exercise (which includes a seven-minute warm-up, four-minute stretch, and a four-minute cooldown), you now have forty-five minutes to devote to the actual workout. What should you do for those forty-five minutes—walk, run on a treadmill, row, lift weights, do a nautilus routine, do some curls?

I'm assuming of course you have all the other factors figured out (lifestyle, medical and orthopedic background, body type, and current level of fitness and motivation). If your goal is to firm and tone, twenty-five to thirty-five minutes should be devoted to anaerobic-type and ten minutes to aerobic exercise. Mondays, Wednesdays, and Fridays can be geared more to firming and toning, and either Tuesdays, Thursdays, Saturdays, or Sundays can be devoted to exercising more aerobically. You can exercise on any or all of these days, depending on your time constraints, goals and type of exercise.

Remember, if your goal is to firm rather than lose weight, energy (intensity) is more important than period (time), so your muscles will need more rest than if you were doing more aerobic exercise. I do recommend resting at least one day per week, regardless of what your fitness goals are. When trying to firm and tone, pay special attention to your body type and to any orthopedic considerations that you may have.

In determining how to allocate time during your workload phase when firming, remember that you want to try to achieve balance throughout your body. You want to create strength and endurance for your upper body, abdominal region, and lower body.

If you choose to lift weights to firm any part of the body, and if you have a tendency to bulk easily or are big and flabby, using low weight and high repetitions is the *only* way you will meet your goals. If you lift more weight, sure you may get firmer, but you'll add size at the same time.

TIP 108

The more weight you use while lifting, the more you will push the fat deposits farther and farther out, creating a very unflattering look. Do not think that the more weight you use the firmer you'll get.

Everyone's body reacts differently to various exercises, but sometimes you may choose the correct exercise and do it incorrectly. That's why you need to experiment more when trying to firm and tone. Because there are so many exercises to choose from, most people just follow the advice of trainers at their local club. The exercises that are recommended are basically the same and usually involve either weight lifting and/or weight machines such as a Nautilus or Cybex circuit. When you read chapter 10, The Ultimate Workout, you will be better able to choose the exercises and workout that work best for you.

If your goal is to firm or tone and you choose to use weights, and if you are of slight build and do not bulk easily, you should do exercises using heavier weights and low to moderate repetitions. You need to build strength as well as endurance. Be careful not to overdo it, though. The more weight you use, the more chance you have of injuring yourself. This is a common mistake made by many, especially you guys out there who want to get "big." It doesn't matter how big you are but rather how strong you are. Big does not mean strong, just as small or slender does not indicate weakness.

Unless you are an athlete who plays a sport requiring enormous bulk and strength, or your job requires it, the majority of Americans do not need and will never use that bulk or strength. Rarely do we use all the strength we try so hard to attain. It's much healthier and beneficial to possess equal strength throughout the body than it is to be able to bench press three hundred pounds.

TIP 109

It's much easier for a heavy or big individual to firm or tone and lose weight than it is to add size and bulk to a thin, light person.

You need to consume tremendous amounts of calories on a very consistent basis to add a lot of natural size to the body. Most people's lifestyles do not allow them to eat many times throughout the entire day. If you want to lose weight and mass or to firm and tone, your diet is important, but exercise is more important. If you overeat one day, you can make up, or better yet burn off those extra calories with either more exercise or more intense exercise.

If you skip or miss meals while trying to add bulk and size, exercise cannot help you. In fact, you could lose mass and size instead of gaining, because you could be burning too many calories during your exercise routine.

The following are the best exercises to firm and tone various parts of your body. The amount of weight, number of repetitions, and duration varies from individual to individual. To learn how to use the proper form for most of these exercises read chapter 10, The Ultimate Workout.

- To firm your chest: dips, chair dips, push-ups, and triceps push-ups
- Arms: curl/straight bar routine and chin-ups
- Abdominals: sit-ups, leg-outs, one-legged leg lifts, leg lifts, elbows to knees and knees to elbows
- Back, shoulders, and lats: curl bar or straight bar routine, pull-ups and chin-ups, dips, upside-down push-ups
- Legs: rope jumping, standing leg-lifts, leg extension and leg curls, vertical scissors on mat
- Hips: standing knee to opposite chest, standing leg lifts to side
- Buttocks and inner thighs: rope jumping, angled knee bends and one-legged angled knee bends, full-bend good mornings, vertical scissors

All these exercises make up your menu. The most important thing to consider before performing any exercise is your medical and orthopedic background first, and body type second. Remember, it does not matter how great the exercise is if you cannot exercise more consistently.

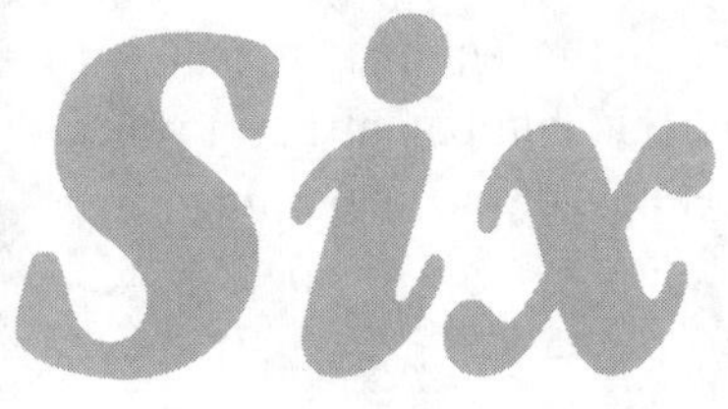

YOUR MINI-GUIDE TO HOME FITNESS EQUIPMENT

OVERVIEW

Before selecting *any* fitness equipment, you must consider the following: Are you really going to use it on a regular basis? If properly used, will the equipment match your fitness needs and goals? Will this equipment harm you orthopedically? The best advice I can give you concerning fitness equipment is this:

TIP 110

If you have a limited budget, buy the best quality fitness equipment you can that falls into your price range; this is especially true with regard to electronic equipment.

True value is largely a function of use. If you spend $1,000 on a treadmill but hardly use it, and your neighbor spends $3,000 on a treadmill and uses it regularly, who made the best investment?

TIP 111

According to a study by *The Wall Street Journal,* 60 to 70 percent of all home fitness equipment purchased is not used after the first six months.

Why? There are many possibilities—lack of knowledge about how to operate it properly, no motivation, breakdown of the equipment itself, lower quality of equipment than expected, not seeing results fast enough, it's noisy, it shakes, it's too big or too small. The list goes on.

I compare someone shopping for fitness equipment to a kid in a large toy store looking for toys. Often fitness equipment purchases are impulsive and therefore not the best decisions. I cannot tell you how many clients I have had who own more fitness equipment than some small retailers. Most Americans today have some piece of unused fitness equipment lying around, perhaps even in use as a clothing hanger.

I believe it is the responsibility of the retailer who sells you the piece of equipment to do everything he or she can to make sure you're properly educated on how to use it. In addition, your retailer has a number of other responsibilities to you, the buyer, including: explaining the basic principles of fitness, determining your fitness goals and how the piece of equipment can help you reach the goals, providing educational and technical support, and acting as a reference to other professionals in the fitness industry.

TIP 112

For those of you tempted to buy intricate fitness equipment from TV, discount stores, department stores, and the like: Be careful! Not only is most of the equipment sold through these mediums cheaply made, but who is going to fix it *when* it breaks down? And yes, it almost always breaks.

The following pages discuss what I feel are the best pieces of fitness equipment manufactured for home use today.

TREADMILL VS. STATIONARY BIKE

Treadmill

Three factors to consider here: space, money, and safety. If *one* or more of these factors does not make sense, then do not buy a treadmill. You need a space approximately six feet by three feet with at least a seven-foot ceiling, and you can plan on spending anywhere from $1,000 to $3,000 for a good quality treadmill.

TIP 113

With treadmills, the motor is the most important element. Motors rated under 2.0 horsepower are at risk of burning out and will not be able to turn the belt safely and smoothly. Additionally, try to purchase a treadmill with side safety rails and a safety key feature.

Although you may burn more calories using a treadmill (depending upon speed and elevation angle), it is more dangerous to use than a bike.

TIP 114

You use more major muscles treadmilling than biking, and treadmilling is a better weight-bearing exercise (especially important for preventing osteoporosis). You also develop more agility, balance, and coordination with a treadmill than a bike.

You can, however, fall off a treadmill and injure yourself. Treadmill workouts are not weather dependent and can be done 24 hours a day, 365 days a year. If properly used and combined with other exercises, the treadmill is a good tool for getting in shape, and can be used for warming up and cooling down.

Stationary Bicycle

Choosing a stationary bike does not require as many purchase decisions as a treadmill. Stationary bikes are usually classified as either manual or electronic. In other words, the tension and resistance can be adjusted either by hand or by pushing a button. Manual bikes have three distinct advantages over the electronic ones. Aside from its lower price, with a manual bike, all you need to do is get on and ride, no fidgeting with gadgets.

TIP 115

The biggest advantage to purchasing a manual bike is that you can decrease the tension to zero, or no resistance.

This is essential for those individuals who do not have the strength to pedal even on the lightest level available on an electronic bike. For certain medical conditions, such as a heart problem, if you pedal with little or no tension, you're able to go for a longer period of time without having to stop. Also, your heart rate may rise too quickly if the tension is too strenuous.

Although electronic bikes are, on average, more expensive, they too have advantages. They offer a greater degree of programming, more options (displays and screens, heart-rate monitors), and more feedback (i.e. calories burned, workload). All of these elements may help motivate a user at first, but long-term motivation comes from within.

It is much safer to warm up on any type of bike, especially a manual one, because you can control the workload better than on a treadmill. Also, if you cannot walk or jog more than 4.0 miles an hour, you can burn more calories riding at high rpm. You do not put the stress on your joints that you do with a treadmill, and it's pretty difficult to fall off a bike.

On the down side, biking is not a great weight-bearing exercise, so you must supplement it with other exercises. You do not develop the coordination, agility, and balance that you would with a treadmill, either.

Caution: most electronic fitness equipment requires batteries, and/or an individual source of electricity (a dedicated circuit), in some cases 220 VAC rather than 110. Make sure you understand the electrical requirements before your purchase.

TIP 116

There are two basic types of exercise bikes: upright and recumbent.

Upright bikes are the more familiar ones, on which you sit in an upright position. Approximately 60 percent of your body is supported, so there is less chance of injuring yourself than on a treadmill. Upright bikes are better suited for individuals who cannot run, who have minor back problems, are very overweight, or have heart conditions. Uprights are also better for certain sport-specific training such as skiing, skating, cycling, and sports in which you use more of your quad muscles (front of thigh) than hamstrings (back of legs).

TIP 117

A recumbent bike is a bike on which you are sitting, but your legs are level with or slightly below your heart when your feet are on the pedals.

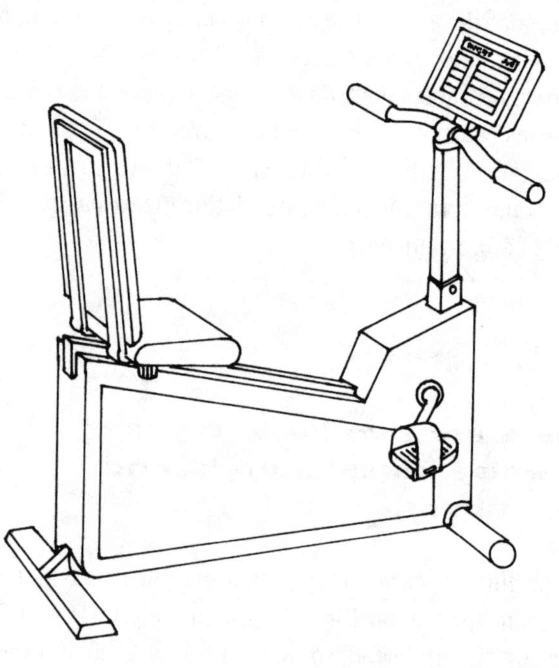

This type of bike has gained tremendous popularity over the past five years. It is no longer used only by the disabled, the elderly, people with severe back, knee, or heart conditions, or very overweight people. More riders are using this bike because it is very comfortable, placing very little stress on the back and knees. Some manufacturers claim that you burn more calories on a recumbent than an upright because it utilizes more muscle groups and you use more energy lifting and keeping your feet on the pedals while exercising. I personally think it is the single best aerobic tool you can purchase if you have any of the above conditions. In addition, if you are elderly or do not like to walk, it can be wonderful in building up your cardiovascular system.

You have even less chance of injury when using the recumbent bike, because you're lower to the ground, and your entire body (except for your arms) is supported throughout your entire ride. It is also the number one aerobic exercise in terms of safety for those with a knee or back condition.

STAIR CLIMBERS, SKI MACHINES, AND ROWERS

Stair Climbers

TIP 118

If you are thinking of buying any one of the many brands of stair climbers, you need to have perfect knees, a perfect back, and no tendency to bulk or add size in your legs, hips, or buttocks.

That should narrow it down to only a small percentage of users, yet stair climber sales have steadily grown throughout the past five years. People buy it and use it because it gives them a "good sweat," and they think it's really good to firm their legs and butts. But after reading up to this point in this book, you now know that's the farthest from the truth.

If you meet the criteria mentioned above, stair climbers are a good tool for rounding out your butt, adding some size to your lower body, and adding some cardiorespiratory benefit to your overall fitness level.

TIP 119

***Caution:* Even if you have good knees and a good back, recent statistics have shown that those who do a lot of stair climbing develop problems in these areas of the body that do not show up or act up until years later, similar to injuries from aerobics classes.**

Most stair climber injuries are caused not by the exercise per se but are mostly due to improper use and form while performing the exercise. For instance, when you lean on your forearms or put too much weight on your hands while stair climbing, you are putting an enormous amount of undue stress on your arms, neck, back, and hands. If you're too darn lazy to do it correctly, why do it at all?

Even though you do not need much room for stair

climbers, I do not highly recommend them. If you're healthy enough to use a stair climber, you're better off actually walking or running up a real staircase and you'll get more fitness benefits this way. Besides, I never met anyone who used stair climbers as their sole aerobic exercise who was truly aerobically fit.

TIP 120

For people who are unfit, stair climbers are not a wise choice to use for warming up or cooling down, since your heart rate could rise too quickly.

Ski Machines

Ski machines provide a wonderful aerobic workout and overall exercise. The problem is that they are so damn hard to use in the beginning. You need to combine coordination, agility, and good balance in addition to having an already good base of aerobic power in order to use them long enough to get results. Most people do not have the attention span to stick to them long enough to reap the fitness benefits. It's a shame, because I think skiing is an excellent form of exercise.

Ski machines do not require a lot of ceiling height but do require at least eight feet in length and two to three feet in width, depending how wide your shoulders are. Skiing does work your upper body a little and is a very low-jarring weight-bearing exercise. It also puts less stress on your lower body than walking or running, but not less than biking.

TIP 121

If you have severe neck problems, steer clear of ski machines.

Using ski machines to get in shape for either downhill or cross-country skiing is excellent. It's okay on the knees and back, and is often used for people with hip problems. If you have the skills and perseverance to use a ski machine, I highly recommend it as an excellent form of aerobic exercise. Used with rope jumping, skiing is perhaps one of the best cardiovascular conditioning programs you can do.

Rowers

Rowing is a decent way to condition your aerobic system, firm your legs and buttocks, and help firm your upper body as well. However, it is important to choose a rower that gives you full range of motion, and unfortunately few do. People with bad knees and bad backs and necks should proceed with caution. However, rowing is a good exercise that also works the abdominals, and as you become more advanced, try to row without hooking your feet under the straps, it will take a lot of stress off your back, legs, neck, and arms.

Rowers take up a lot of length—you need about eight or ten feet to work comfortably—but you are low to the ground, so it is pretty hard to injure yourself seriously.

Rowing is a very good way to develop upper body muscular endurance, and the good rowers have a wide variety of tension selections that allow you to grow into it. I do recommend using a rower if you want to add to your fitness level in conjunction with other exercises.

Please note: for an unfit person, even though rowing is considered aerobic, do not use it for warming up or cooling down, because your heart rate tends to rise more quickly than with other exercises previously mentioned.

You may or may not experience some of the conditions that I state, or you may develop some other side effects. Remember to listen to your body while using any of the fitness equipment mentioned above, or any others.

FREE WEIGHTS, SELECTORIZED WEIGHT MACHINES

This section is difficult to explain and will be one of the toughest to understand fully because there are so many ways to exercise using weights. Each way has a certain technique when properly performed and can help you achieve fitness, but methods vary widely in complexity from one form to another. Whether you do a Universal circuit, or use free weights, all forms can be classified as weight lifting. When you move an object, including your own body, by lifting it to the side, above, behind, or you pull or push that object, you are in a sense lifting a weight. Bodybuilding is a sport that utilizes one, some, or hopefully many techniques of weight lifting.

Which is better: using free weights, doing a thirty-minute weight circuit, or lifting your own body weight up and down?

TIP 123

When choosing to buy any fitness equipment in general, and weight equipment in particular, the number one factor to consider is your medical and orthopedic background.

Your background is going to dictate which type of stress your body can take without harm. More people injure themselves while lifting weights than perhaps any other type of exercising, and many injuries can be serious. If you fall off your treadmill and break your ankle, your ankle will eventually heal. But if you blow out your shoulder or tear a muscle weight lifting, chances are you'll have problems for the rest of your life. That is the main reason why I do not believe in weight lifting for *any* child under the age of sixteen, and even then, always with professional supervision.

Remember our little discussion on strength training versus endurance training? Assuming you have a full understanding of what your body should and should not be doing, and your goals are defined, next you must consider how much time you will have to devote to your strengthening or endurance training. The more complex and varied numbers of weights or machines you choose, the more time you'll need to work out.

TIP 124

If you are pressed for time, do not choose free weights, because it takes longer to train with them—changing weights, changing bars—and you need another person commonly referred to as a spotter.

It's always wise to have a spotter, especially when just starting out with weights, to ensure you don't hurt yourself with certain exercises, such as the bench press and behind the neck press.

If time is not a factor, a free weight workout done properly is one of the most effective ways to build your strength or endurance. It is more natural than using a machine, because it closely simulates what you do in real life—pushing, pulling, etc. However, technique is critical.

You need an area at least ten feet by ten feet to fully stock your home with free weights, and you can easily use up to another 100 square feet, if you want to really impress your friends.

TIP 125

Don't purchase free weights if you do not have enough room for both you and a spotter to move around comfortably.

You can purchase either a standard 1¼-inch-diameter weight bar and weights (for lighter use), or Olympic-style weights (2 inches in diameter), which are better for using weights over 100 lbs. Also, the benches and other accessories come in either standard or Olympic style.

"Selectorized" weight machines offer a wide range of options and are much safer to exercise with. You do however need at least a seven by seven area with seven-foot ceilings or higher. But their use does not require a spotter, they are more "user friendly," you have less chance for injury, your form is more controlled, and they're very practical for the disabled, the elderly, and people with orthopedic constraints. You can circuit train and move faster through your workout, and there's no changing of weights other than selecting a different amount by moving a pin to do so.

On the down side, weight machines are somewhat pricey, do not give you a full range of motion, are dangerous if children have access to them, and do not allow you to develop a "pure" strength as you can with free weights or other exercise techniques.

I rate selectorized weight machines as a moderately good way to strengthen your body. One distinct advantage over free weights is that some brands offer an excellent way to develop good leg strength by performing leg extensions and leg curls, which is the single best exercise to help protect and rehab your knees, especially if you ski or play basketball, football, or tennis.

MISCELLANEOUS EQUIPMENT

There are more fitness equipment manufacturers popping up every day in the never-ending search for the ultimate exercise, which, quite honestly, is hurting the industry as a whole. The cheaper the quality, the cheaper the consumer can purchase it for. And, unfortunately, the average consumer does not know enough to make an educated decision on his or her own. In real estate, you need to know only three words—location, location, location. With fitness equipment and exercise it's reliability, reliability, reliability.

TIP 126

If you really want to build "pure" muscle strength and endurance, I highly recommend buying a chin-up/dip unit.

A good chin-up/dip unit takes at least eight or nine feet of ceiling height to accommodate a unit that will allow you to perform chins or pulls without having to bend your legs underneath you. Most units are approximately seven feet high and three feet wide. These are not very expensive, but if you're over five feet six, you will not be able to perform exercises without feeling constricted.

Benefits: Full range of motion, easy on your joints, gives you a more natural look, elongates muscles, does not require a lot of time for a full upper body workout, and unlike free weights or machines, can easily be simulated. Great for building power and strength, especially when you add weights to your body while doing your reps.

TIP 127

You are less likely to injure yourself while performing chin-ups and dips than exercising with free weights.

Downside: It's difficult to lift your body up and down, especially for women; when starting out, you may need a spotter. Additionally, the less expensive models are not well constructed or durable.

Other Recommended Fitness Equipment

Jump ropes, weighted and unweighted, for aerobic and full-body toning. Dumbbells for upper body isolating, strength and endurance training. Hand grips for strengthening hands, wrists, and forearms. Stationary bikes with an air-dyne, because the fan helps cool the body. An aerobic bar, used for stretching, toning, and firming hips, buttocks, and thighs. A curl bar and straight bar, used for firming and toning the entire body. A firm nonbending exercise mat, for stretching, abdominal exercises, and literally hundreds of exercises for the entire body. Heart-rate monitors, to gauge and consistently monitor your heart rate during exercise, are especially useful for exercisers with a heart condition. A wooden board for rope jumping to help absorb shock to the body. A simple exercise bench to use for lifting, and strengthening abdominal muscles. These are a few pieces of fitness equipment and accessories I feel can add to your fitness level.

TIP 128

It's important to note that there is *no* one piece of fitness equipment that can get you totally fit in and by itself.

However, if I had to choose one piece of fitness equipment that would be the most effective, it would be, without hesitation, a jump rope.

TIP 129

The best piece of fitness equipment to purchase is one that works in a safe, effective, and efficient manner and fits within your budget.

RECOMMENDED BUYS

- Best electronic upright bike: Lifecycle 6500 HR
  Price range: $1,200–$1,600
- Best manual bike:
  One user: Schwinn 105P
  Price range: $350–$400
  Many users: Schwinn DX900
  Price range: $1,000–$1,200
- Best electronic recumbent bike: Lifecycle 5500 R
  Price range: $1,500–$2,000
- Best rowers: Concept II Rower and Water Rower
  Price range: $750–$895 and $1,295–$1,695
- Best treadmill: Trotter CXT Plus
  Price range: $2,700–$3,600
  (Note: This is the only treadmill manufacturer that provides a three-year parts and labor warranty.)
- Best free weight manufacturer for both Olympic and standard:
  One user (private): Tuff Stuff (both Olympic and standard)
  Price range: $100–$1,400
  Many users (commercial): Trotter and Paramount (both Olympic and standard)
  Price range: $300–$3,000 (extra options)
- Best home unit selectorized weight machine: Paramount PFC
  Price range: $2,500 (standard unit) to $4,000 (extra options)
- Best large home unit selectorized weight machine: Paramount FTX

Price range: $3,400 (basic units) to $5,000 (extra options)

- Best stair climber:
  One user (private): Climbmax PC
  Price range: $1,900–$2,200
  Many users (commercial): Climbmax
  Price range: $2,000–$3,000

I've conducted business ventures with some of the country's biggest and best retailers of fitness equipment. *No one* holds a candle to Core Fitness Management, located in Southampton, New York, 1–800–510–3190. They ship and deliver fitness equipment around the world and can personally service any piece of equipment from Florida to Maine. There are no excuses with this company: they deliver on time, rent and lease both home and commercial equipment, design home gyms, hotel and corporate facilities, health clubs, spas, condos and co-ops. You name it, Core Fitness Management can do it.

Seven

ACHES AND PAINS

What are you supposed to do immediately after spraining an ankle or straining your hamstring? A good way to remember what steps you should take to get yourself back to 100 percent is to learn this simple acronym—PRICE.

P = PROTECT your body and more specifically, the body part that's injured, from further injury. If you continue to exercise when you get hurt, you're only asking for trouble.

The first and foremost rule on preventing further damage while performing *any* exercise or sport is that if a part of your body is hurting, stop immediately. It doesn't make you less of a person to walk off the tennis or basketball court because you twisted your ankle.

TIP 130

Ceasing exercise is the first phase in treating an athletic-related injury.

Following are common exercises and activities, and the body parts they usually affect most:

- Aerobics classes, step classes, stair climbers—knees, ankles, back, feet, shins, calves
- Basketball—ankles, knees, calves, head, eyes
- Downhill skiing—knees, ankles, back, head
- Golf—back, forearms, upper arms, hips
- Horseback riding—back, hips, knees, legs
- Running/jogging—ankles, knees, back, heel, calves, feet, shins, hips, front and rear thighs
- Softball—shoulders, ankles, knees
- Racquet sports—eyes, head, rear thighs, groin, calves, feet

- Rope jumping—calves, back
- Rowing—knees, back
- Tennis—calves, groin, rear thighs
- Touch football—ankles, knees, calves, rear thighs
- Weight lifting—neck, back, hips, feet, front and rear thighs, shoulders
- Yoga—strained and torn muscles throughout body
- Walking—back, knees

If you are susceptible to certain injuries, please take extra precaution while playing any sport or engaging in any exercise.

TIP 131

Most injuries occur because of lack of proper warm-up and stretching beforehand, or because of poor fitness levels.

The next phase in treating yourself for injury is REST. Rest does not mean walking it off. You cannot and will not walk off a sprained ankle or a strained muscle. It requires, among other things, immediate rest. Rest also means to rest until it is just about completely healed. Isn't it better to rest your calf a couple of days after injuring it, than to risk pulling or tearing it and missing the next six to twelve weeks?

Next on the list is ICE. Take a plastic bag, put ten to twenty ice cubes in it, and tie it. Put it in another bag to prevent leakage. Then apply the bag directly to the injury with a 5-inch ace bandage so it does not fall off. Apply for stints of twenty to forty minutes, twice a day, until all the swelling or major pain has subsided. If it takes you five days to heal, then apply ice for five days.

TIP 132

Do not apply heat after any injury. If you are not sure what to do, ask your doctor or local pharmacist.

Next we have COMPRESSION—not just compression with the ice, but also after icing, making sure that the injury is sufficiently wrapped with the right amount of pressure. Not too light and not too heavy.

Compression allows the swelling to dissipate more quickly than just laying the ice bag on the injury. I cannot overemphasize the importance of icing and compression after an injury.

Finally, ELEVATE. Make sure that while you are icing, sleeping, resting, watching TV, or reading, the body part that is injured is elevated. This allows the blood to flow more smoothly to the injured area.

There is no substitution for the PRICE system. Do not ignore the fact that you're injured. Everybody hurts themselves at some point.

TIP 133

The most important thing to remember when you injure yourself is to ice and rest long enough for your injury to heal.

If you are not sure what to do after getting hurt, ask a doctor who is familiar with your type of injury. Obviously, the best way to protect yourself against injury is to become fit before going out there and playing *any* sport.

TIP 134

Stay away from exercises or sports that you know aggravate parts of your body where you are weak or have orthopedic problems.

If you are going to take an exercise class or go out and play hoops, first weigh the benefits against the risks. Just because you used to be in great shape and went out and dominated a particular sport ten or more years ago, don't think your body will respond in the same way today, especially if you've not kept up with a conditioning program.

Another common mistake made by many who exercise is that they exercise out of their heart rate zone. Your heart cannot take the stress in most cases, so be especially careful in very hot or very cold climates. Inexperience can get you into trouble as well. If you do not know where to position yourself on a tennis court when playing tennis doubles, don't be shocked when you have ball marks on the backs of your legs by the end of your tennis day. The older you are, the more risk you have for skeletal injuries. And if you have a special medical condition, make sure there is a medical facility nearby if you're engaging in any vigorous activity.

Muscle soreness, especially when beginning an exercise program, is quite common. However, if you cannot get out of bed the next day, you definitely overdid it. But if you wake up and your body feels slightly sore, then you did just the right amount of exercise. In a week or less, this soreness will dissipate. If it does not, check with your doctor. Warming up, stretching, and cooling down help prevent muscle soreness.

Most people know when there is something wrong with their body. Listen to it. Nine out of ten times you're right. Do not ignore warning signals when exercising. The pain will not go away, it will only get worse. On the other hand, if you turn your ankle, rest a day or so, but start getting back into your exercise regimen by biking, stretching, and performing any exercise that does not inflame the ankle. If you work out the rest of your body while injured, you will heal faster, because the body is sending signals to the injured area. In addition, atrophy will not set in as fast.

TIP 135

Learn to distinguish muscle fatigue from sharp pain.

Muscle fatigue is a general feeling of fatigue throughout the entire muscle that you've been exercising. The muscle may feel sore and/or tight. Pain, however, will be a more localized, intense sensation. If you're doing sit-ups and your stomach muscles feel tired and tight, keep going a little bit more. But if you get a sharp, stabbing pain after just one or two repetitions, stop and consult with a professional. Confusing muscle fatigue with pain can lead to injury. It's a tough thing to distinguish, especially for beginning exercisers. If you're not sure how to perform an exercise, seek advice from someone within the fitness industry.

TIP 136

Do not ask your friends for advice on exercise and fitness or what you should do if you have injured yourself.

When in doubt, ask a professional—be it exercise or, for that matter, any subject that you're not sure what steps are needed to take to ensure safety, proper form, and technique. Which would you prefer, to not ask and get hurt, or to ask, learn, and never injure yourself? For some strange reason, people are very shy about exercise;

they think it's dumb to ask. Fitness is an art. You need to study it and gain experience in any field of fitness to be an expert. It's no different from being a plumber, accountant, lawyer, or doctor. So, the next time you're hesitant to ask, throw away your ego and do it. Only a fool doesn't ask what he or she doesn't know.

Proper footwear and clothing are also helpful in preventing injuries and overheating. Go out and spend some money on the right apparel. If your plumber showed up with carpenter's tools, could he do an effective job? Wear clothes that breathe, preferably cotton. There are more sports shops and sneaker outlets today than one can count. Go in, find and ask the most knowledgeable person for advice. And when a couple of them from different stores agree with one another, then make the right purchase.

Eight

BAD BACK BLUES

It's generally difficult to determine what exercises are particularly good or bad for the back. My theory on why the back is so mysterious when it comes to exercise, and its reaction to exercise, is that because it is a very large region of the body, we sometimes think we've injured our back but have hurt another part of our body that is close by. Because of this, it is often hard to isolate pain or discomfort that can be accurately described as back-related.

Just because you read or hear that an exercise is good or bad for your back, does not necessarily mean it's good or bad for you. While it's true that certain exercises are categorized as contraindicative (should be avoided), most exercises have not been proven to be harmful. There are many misconceptions regarding exercises and back care. For instance, the health club that you just joined did not tell you that doing a step class would probably aggravate your lower back pain, did they? Or that performing bent-knee sit-ups could help strengthen your back, if done correctly? The point here is that what may be good for me, may not be good for you, or vice versa.

Of all the people I've consulted with over the years regarding *any* type of back problem, nine out of ten had poor flexibility, especially in their hamstrings and torso areas. Which makes sense, since most activities, sports and exercises put stress on these areas of your body. But as their flexibility increased their back pain *decreased.* It's important to note, however, that it's not just stretching that helps, it's *how* one stretches that makes a difference.

Stress to the back region is caused by: inactivity, not properly warming up and stretching before exercising or playing sports, not strengthening abdominals and increasing hamstring flexibility while exercising, and improper exercise.

TIP 137

Stretching is the most important phase of anyone's workout.

BACK PAIN, INJURIES, AND EXERCISE

Dr. Joseph M. Flagello, a chiropractic physician in Palm Beach, Florida, reports that sprains and strains are the most common back injuries. He estimates that only 20 to 30 percent of those who injure themselves are fit, which happens to be close to the national average.

TIP 138

There is a direct correlation between lack of fitness and back problems. Muscles are designed to provide primary stability for the joints. The effects of exercise are the development or improvement of strength, endurance, cardiovascular fitness, mobility, flexibility, relaxation, coordination, and skill.

Among professionals, Wolf's Law states that bones model according to imposed demands. In other words, form follows function. Therefore, it is obvious that it is important to exercise and put stress and demands on the musculoskeletal system. Of course this must be within the patient's limits, because repeated and undue stress will cause pain and dysfunction.

TIP 139

People who are unfit and don't exercise are more prone to low back pain and other orthopedic problems.

The adage "An ounce of prevention is worth a pound of cure" is as applicable here as anywhere else.

In some cases, tight hamstrings will tend to tilt the pelvis posteriorly. This in turn "flattens out" the normal lumbar lordosis (C-shaped curve of the spine as viewed from the side). Contact sports tend to create the most opportunities for injury.

Improper technique in any sport such as weight lifting, running, racquetball, etc. may cause injury. Golf, even with proper form, may tend to create a back problem or aggravate a preexisting condition by the nature of the golf swing.

Slipped discs are very common injuries. Put simply, a disc is a shock-absorbing sponge located between two vertebral bodies in a person's spine. It consists of a wide rim of cartilage that surrounds a soft, water-absorbent nucleus. The strips of cartilage are strong and arranged like layers of an onion. The nucleus distributes pressure hydrostatically or equally in all directions. This allows the joint to bear considerable amounts of weight. Physicians may refer to a slipped disc as one that is bulging or actually herniated. A protruding disc or bulging disc will cause pain when the strips of cartilage (called annular fibers) have a deficit that permits the nucleus to bulge farther than its normal degree. In a disc that is herniated the nucleus will actually burst through the annular fibers.

TIP 140

When it comes to prescribing rehabilitative exercises for back pain and injuries, it is very difficult to make general recommendations.

The doctor needs to determine, on a case by case basis, the type of protrusion and how best to strengthen the surrounding musculature. A doctor will usually consult with the patient's physical therapist in order to determine the best treatment.

TIP 141

Any exercise that creates lateralizing pain, which is pain that shoots out from the center into the leg or buttock, is a contraindicated exercise and therefore should be eliminated from your routine.

If the pain becomes more localized or centralized, then it is usually okay to continue with that exercise or group of exercises, provided that the pain dissipates and soon goes completely away.

There are two existing treatments that doctors follow for rehabilitation. They seem to contradict one another, yet both are successful. One advocates extension exercises and the other advocates flexion exercises. An example of an extension exercise is a back bend, in which the involved joint angles are increasing. An example of a flexion exercise is a sit-up, in which the involved joint angles are decreasing. Trial and error determines what therapy is best for the patient.

TIP 142

Determining centralization of pain is the single most important guide you have in choosing the correct exercises for your problem.

Initial pain increase during rehabilitative exercises is common and can be expected. The pain should quickly diminish at least to its former level. This usually occurs during the first exercise session and then centralizes. If a patient has significant lower back pain when lying in bed and cannot move without experiencing pain, then rehab exercises should be cautious and unhurried.

TIP 143

Do not continue with an exercise if symptoms are much worse immediately after exercising and remain worse the next day or if, during exercising, symptoms are produced or increased in the leg below the knee.

Contrary to popular belief, sit-ups are not bad for everyone's back. The ability to do a curled-trunk sit-up should be considered a normal accomplishment. People should be able to get up easily from a supine position without having to roll over on the side or push themselves up with their arms.

Abdominal strength and endurance play an important role in the prevention of low back pain. Low back problems are caused by many factors such as structural abnormalities, disease, accidents, poor posture or lifting mechanics, failure to warm up prior to exercise, and lack of flexibility and muscular strength and endurance in the midtrunk area. Many of these problems can be prevented by using appropriate lifting techniques and good posture; warming up and stretching before exercising; increasing midtrunk strength, endurance, and flexibility.

TIP 144

While normal flexibility of the back is desirable, excessive flexibility is not, nor does it guarantee a pain-free back.

The people most in danger of being adversely affected by repeated sit-ups with knees bent are children and youths, because they are more apt to hyperextend since they have more flexibility than adults. Done to excess, sit-ups may increase the tendency toward developing a round upper back and forward shoulders.

I'm frequently asked whether holding the feet down while performing a sit-up causes any problem with one's back. Assuming that abdominal strength is normal, the answer is that it might not if one is performing only a few sit-ups, but it can make a great deal of difference if many repetitions are performed. With repeated sit-ups, an individual's abdominal muscles may fatigue, causing the lower back to arch. This occurs because hip flexor endurance is greater than abdominal endurance. If an individual's feet are being held down, this transition may go unnoticed.

Emphasis has been placed on doing sit-ups in a bent-knee position, which automatically flexes the hips in the supine position. When there is weakness in either or both muscle groups involved in the curled-trunk sit-up (abdominal and hip flexor muscles), efforts should be made to correct the weakness and restore the ability to perform the movement correctly. Using the sit-up exercise to try to correct the abdominal weakness is a mistake, because when marked weakness exists, the hip flexors initiate and perform the movement with the low back hyperextended.

Posture

TIP 145

We spend the majority of our time either sleeping, sitting, or standing. Therefore it is important to consider posture in all three positions.

Here are some helpful points to be aware of: avoid extremes in your posture; a small pillow placed at the lowest part of your back (just above the hips) when you are sitting or lying can maintain the normal lower back curve. Avoid military-type positions, which are very rigid, and hyperextension such as locked knees, and head and shoulders pressed back. Avoid standing for prolonged periods of time, as this fatigues the muscles that support the trunk.

In order to improve posture and prevent low back problems increase muscular strength, endurance, and flexibility in the midtrunk region. Remember, muscular imbalance can cause postural deviations, so strengthening the body's musculature evenly is key.

Concentrate on increasing abdominal strength and endurance, increasing flexibility particularly in the lower back and upper legs (hamstrings), and doing plenty of static stretching in order to increase your range of motion gradually.

Muscle Tears

Heavy weight lifting tends to place stress on the body's joints over time, and if the surrounding tendon isn't as strong as the muscle, the muscle may tear, causing the tendon to give out. A certain amount of muscle tear, however, is necessary in order to foster new muscle growth. The vertebrae in the back can handle incredible compressive loading force so long as there is no rotational force or lateral wedging. Consequently, proper form when weight lifting is crucial. Genetics also plays a role in determining how prone an individual is to injury.

RECOMMENDED BACK STRETCHES AND EXERCISES

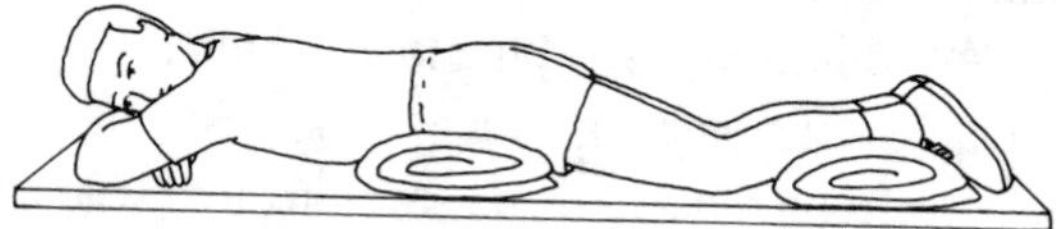

Low back stretching #1: Lying facedown, place a firm pillow under the abdomen and a rolled blanket under the ankles.

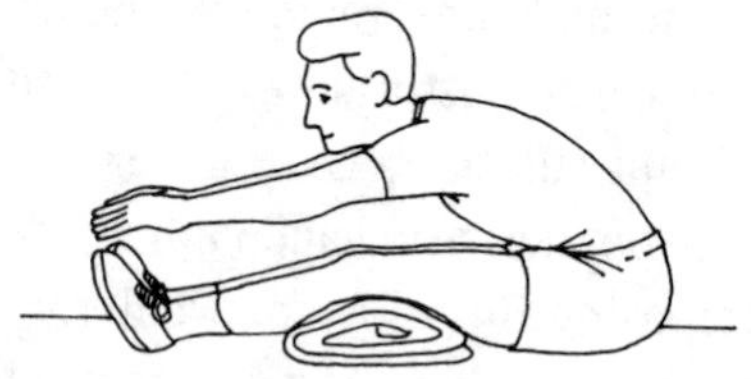

Low back stretching #2: Sit with legs extended forward. Place a rolled blanket under the knees to allow a slight bend in the knees. Pull in with the abdominal muscles, keep the pelvis tilted back, and reach forward toward the toes.

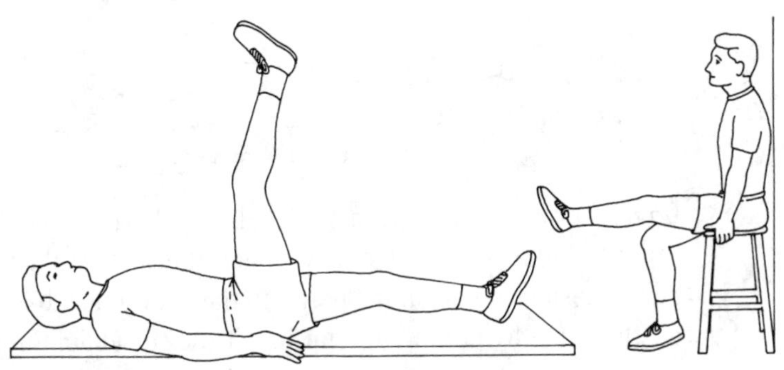

Hamstring stretching: To stretch tight hamstrings, lie supine with legs extended, hold left leg down, and gradually raise the right with the knee straight. To stretch left hamstrings, apply the same procedures to the left leg. Or raise the leg and rest the heel against the back of a chair or other support with hamstrings in stretched position. Or sit on a stool with back against a wall. Keep back straight and buttocks against the wall. With one knee bent, straighten the other.

Hip flexor stretching: To stretch left hip flexors, lie supine with left lower leg hanging over end of table. Pull right knee firmly toward chest to help press low back flat down on table. Keeping low back flat, stretch left hip flexors by pulling the right thigh

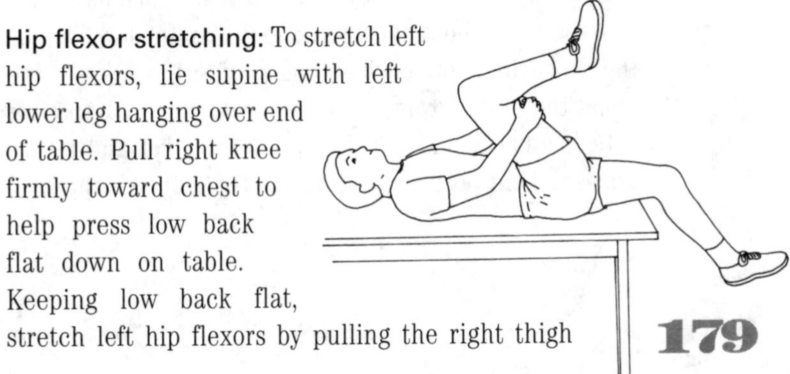

downward toward the table by contracting the buttock muscle. To stretch right hip flexors, lie with the right knee bent hanging over the end of the table, pull left knee toward the chest, and stretch the left thigh.

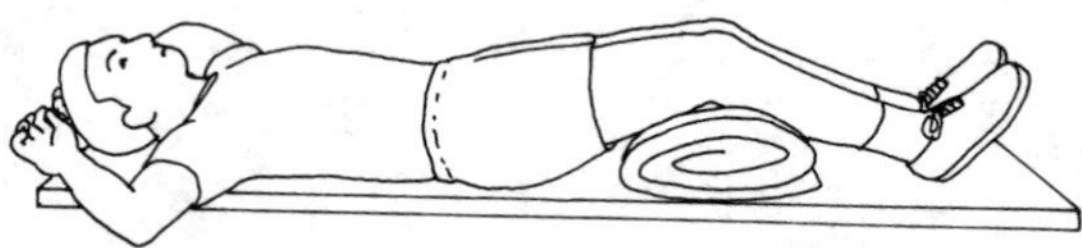

Lower abdominal exercise #1: Lying down, place a rolled blanket or small pillow under the knees. Place hands beside the head, tilt pelvis to flatten the low back on the table by pulling up and in with lower abdominal muscles. Hold low back flat and breathe in and out easily, relaxing the upper abdominal muscles.

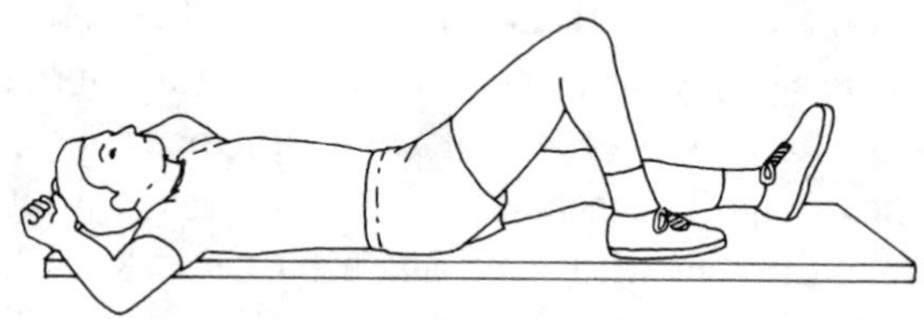

Lower abdominal exercise #2: Lie down on your back with knees bent and feet flat on the mat. Place hands beside the head and tilt the pelvis to flatten the low back on the mat. Hold low back flat and slide the heels down along the mat. Straighten the legs as much as possible with low back held flat. Keep low back flat and return knees to bent position, sliding one leg back at a time.

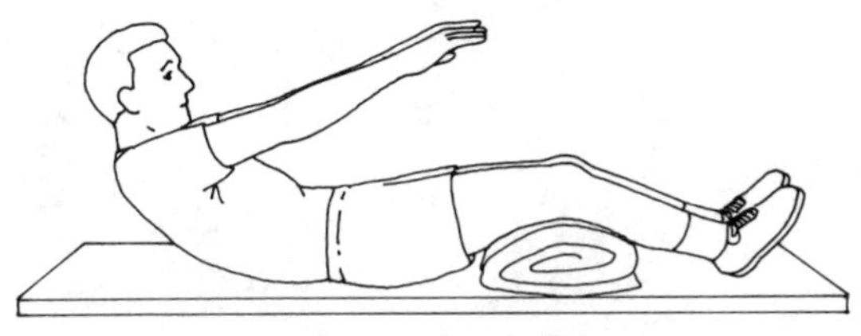

Upper abdominal exercise: Lying down on your back, tilt the pelvis to flatten the low back on the mat. With arms extended forward, raise head and shoulders about eight inches up from the mat.

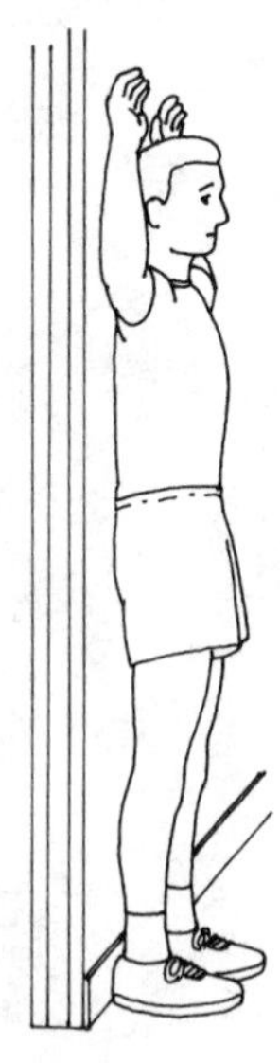

Standing postural exercise: Stand with the back against a wall, heels about three inches from the wall. Place hands up beside head with elbows touching the wall. Tilt pelvis to flatten low back against the wall by pulling the lower abdominal muscles up and in.

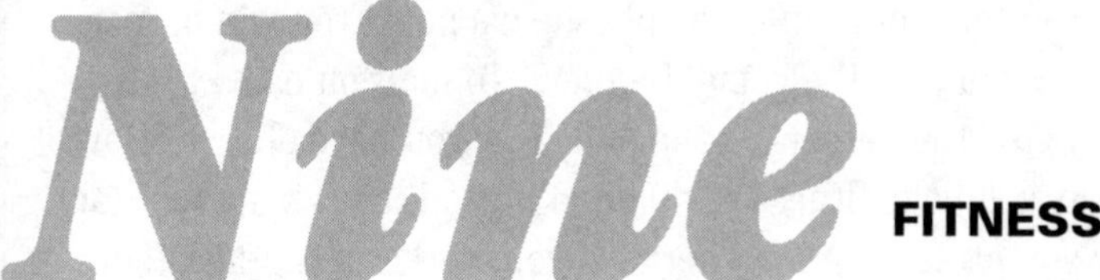

FITNESS STRATEGIES FOR SPECIAL POPULATIONS

Most health problems that develop over the course of one's life are due to either leading a sedentary life or exercising improperly. If you were to bet on a horse race, would you consider a fat, out of shape, low-energy horse to even cross the finish line? The thought of that horse winning *never* enters your mind. People say it's not if you win or lose, it's how you play the game. Baloney! To me, you can *only* win if you give 100 percent in the endeavor you have chosen. How you attack your fitness regimen is a good measuring tool for how you attack life in general. If you work out halfheartedly, it's more than likely you'll do other things the same way. Don't go through the motions of exercise. You will derive more pleasure from exercise if you approach it each time with passion and intensity.

If you have a physical handicap, or you are recovering from a heart attack, or you have high blood pressure, or whatever your present physical condition is, you have all the more reason to engage in a regular fitness program.

TIP 146

Don't use the fact that you're not 100 percent physically as an excuse not to exercise. In fact, in most cases, the only way to get closer to that 100 percent, is to be regular with the proper fitness program.

Drugs, therapy, and the like are a short-term fix. And remember, as always, consult with your physician before starting any fitness program.

HIGH BLOOD PRESSURE (HYPERTENSION)

Hypertension is excessive pressure against artery walls.

- 140/90 is considered the threshold of high blood pressure.
  140 = systolic = force generated against artery walls at contraction.
  90 = diastolic = force generated against artery walls at relaxation.
- One out of four Americans has it.
- Many of the 35 million Americans in this country with high blood pressure take medicine to help protect them from developing a heart attack or stroke.
- The best medications to treat high blood pressure in regular exercisers are clondine (brand name Catapres), methyldopa (Aldomet), and prazosin (Minipress). These prescription medications do not affect heart or muscle function during exercise.
- Beta blockers such as propranolol (Inderal) cause muscle tiredness and weakness and may limit the amount of exercise you can do. For this reason, the intensity level factor of a workout must be milder than normal.
- Check with your doctor for the best course of treatment.
- If you use exercise with other methods of lowering your blood pressure, be careful about participating in sports or activities that require you to hold your breath

when contracting your muscles (i.e. swimming underwater longer than ten seconds, weight lifting, a hard tennis serve). Holding your breath causes pressure in blood vessels to rise to very high levels (300/240 as compared to the normal 120/80).

- Erratic, ballistic exercises can also be dangerous. Sudden bursts of activity can cause irregular heartbeats. Avoid isometric exercises and heavy weight lifting.

TIP 147

Too many people use high blood pressure as a reason not to exercise. Little do they know that with proper exercise, most can lower their medication or even eliminate taking it, *if* they are consistent with their exercise regimen.

Having high blood pressure is a good reason to start a fitness program. In fact, nothing will ever lower your blood pressure as effectively and naturally as exercise.

TIP 148

Although you may be afraid of exercising after you've had a heart attack, exercise can reduce your chances of getting a second attack.

- Exercise will also help you lose weight, increase endurance, elevate your mood, and resume a normal lifestyle.
- Make sure your doctor says you have recovered enough to resume exercising.
- Start by taking an electrocardiogram. This test can predict how much exercise a patient's heart can tolerate. Exercising at 100 bpm for thirty minutes, three times per week (never on successive days) is the recommended exercise prescription.
- STOP if you feel pain or get too tired.
- Symptoms that mean STOP:

  Chest tightness or pain
  Lack of muscle coordination
  Shortness of breath
  Irregular heartbeat
  Fainting
  Tiredness
  Lightheadedness, dizziness

- Symptoms that mean you may have done too much:
  Inability to sleep at night
  Extreme fatigue
  Muscle soreness
  Nausea
  Muscle cramps

TIP 149

A doctor's care and the monitoring of your heart rate during exercising is a must for all heart attack patients.

I recommend wearing a heart-rate monitor while exercising. It can alert you if you are nearing your maximum heart rate (220 minus your age), as well as help you stay in your zone while exercising. What's important to note here is that it's impossible to say how much and how hard one should be exercising after a heart attack. Each case is unique. Only your doctor, ideally the doctor who has been treating you throughout, has the most accurate knowledge regarding these and other factors to consider if you are to engage in an exercise program.

- Before the diabetic begins an exercise program, he or she should undergo a thorough physical examination.
- Types of diabetes:

  Type I: juvenile (insulin dependent diabetes)
  Insufficient production of insulin by pancreas.

  Type II: adult onset
  Insulin is produced but cellular tissues do not respond. Can be controlled through diet, exercise, and oral medication.

TIP 150

Exercise promotes entry of insulin into the cells.

Diabetics engaged in exercise should always have a carbohydrate snack on hand. Other precautions diabetics should take before engaging in an exercise program include checking their urine for the presence of *ketones.* Ketones are by-products of fat metabolism that accumulate in the bloodstream and pass into the urine. Exercising with ketones in the bloodstream can cause nausea, muscle weakness, headaches, and digestive problems.

To test for the presence of ketones, use testing paper called Ketostix (available over the counter at pharmacies). Dip it into the urine. Wait a few seconds. If the paper turns purple, ketones are present and you should not exercise. You may exercise safely if ketones are absent, except in rare cases.

Be alert for signs of low blood-sugar levels during a workout:

- Rapid heartbeat
- Hunger
- Cold sweat
- Shaky all over

If these symtoms occur, STOP EXERCISING immediately and ingest a simple carbohydrate snack or drink (i.e., candy, fruit juice).

Most people who develop diabetes after the age of forty can control their blood-sugar level without taking insulin. How?

- Maintain normal weight
- Eat very little fatty foods
- Eat fiber-rich foods
- Exercise regularly

Being overweight reduces the number of insulin receptors in the body. Cells must have enough receptors for sugar to enter them. If they do not, then the cells are less responsive to insulin.

Those over thirty-five should have an electrocardiogram included in their checkup, because diabetics are at risk for cardiovascular disease.

And always check with your physician to make sure you're following a comprehensive program of exercise, diet, and weight control that's appropriate for you—one that is effective enough to control diabetes, so you can stop taking insulin.

TIP 151

Exercise is one of the best ways to control diabetes because it helps increase the number of insulin receptors.

PHYSICAL DISABILITIES

Research has shown that the physically handicapped can achieve the same physical and emotional benefits from exercise as those who are not disabled.

How to arrange your own exercise program:

- Warm-up and Stretch (5–10 minutes) should include rhythmic, slow stretching movements of the trunk and limb muscles. This increases blood flow and stretches the postural muscles, preparing the body for sustained activity.
- Workload (30 minutes)—During this phase, the cardiovascular system is stressed by aerobic activity.
- Cooldown (5–10 minutes) Allows bodily functions to return to normal.

There are athletic organizations for the disabled that can provide specific workouts; exercises as well as warm-up and cooldown, which include calisthenics; and exercises for:

upper limb disabled
lower limb disabled

upper and lower limb disabled

Here are a few organizations:

- National Handicapped Sports and Recreation Association
  4105 East Florida Avenue, 3rd Floor
  Denver, CO 80222
- National Wheelchair Athletic Association
  40-24 62nd Street
  Woodside, NY 11377
  (718) 424-2929
- American Coalition of Citizens with Disabilities
  1346 Connecticut Avenue, NW
  Washington, DC 20036
- Special Olympics
  1701 K Street, NW, Suite 203
  Washington, DC 20006

For outdoor wheelchair sports, manufacturers have designed removable arms and swinging or removable footrests. Being in a wheelchair is no reason not to be physically fit. You can effectively get your heart rate up to 100 beats per minute and more, which is what you need to strengthen your heart, by exercising with your arms continuously for at least ten minutes. Push the wheels of your wheelchair. If you do this indoors, you can have an extra-wide treadmill custom-made. If you do this outdoors, make sure you stay on level ground. Exercise until your arms feel heavy and fatigued. Wait forty-eight hours and resume in between exercise periods.

A machine called an Upper Body Ergometer (UBE) allows a person sitting in a wheelchair to get aerobic benefits and improve cardiovascular conditioning. It's designed especially for those individuals who cannot use their lower bodies. Cybex and Quinton manufacture these UBEs. Ask your local sporting retailer for a brochure and prices.

Also for arms:

- Arm pulleys: Two basic types. One attaches to the wall. The other attaches to a pole so you don't need to drill a hole. Start with ten minutes and build to thirty minutes, then increase weight of the pulley.
- Punching bag: work up to thirty minutes of continuous punching every other day. Position yourself close enough to the bag, but not too close for it to rebound and hit you back.

The most effective anaerobic upper body workout you can do in a wheelchair is five to ten minutes of exercises with either a 10-lb. curl bar or 15-lb. straight bar. By performing exercises with either one of these bars, you will strengthen your entire upper body but put little stress on your joints (see chapter 10 for correct technique).

TIP 152

Balance, coordination, and agility are often overlooked with anyone's fitness program, especially the handicapped.

I cannot overemphasize how improving your balance, coordination, and agility will not only improve your fitness level but will also help in doing your everyday chores. For those who need to improve in any of these areas, write to me (my address is at the back of the book), and I'll be glad to send you some exercises.

FITNESS AFTER FIFTY

TIP 153

I know fifty-year-olds, sixty-year-olds, and—yes—seventy-year-olds who are more fit than most of the teenagers of today.

Reaching fifty or older doesn't mean life stops. In fact, for many, it is an age at which they're more apt to start a fitness program. When beginning a program, please be careful and don't try to undo fifty or more years in a week or even a month.

TIP 154

The wonderful thing about exercise is that after one year of exercising, the body reacts as if it has been exercising its entire life! Now, that's *power.*

Before embarking on your program, be sure to get a thorough medical examination, including an electrocardiogram. Remember, the basis of physical fitness in later years is a fit cardiovascular system. A good exercise regimen should include three basic components:

- Endurance exercises to condition the heart, lungs, and blood vessels and to induce relaxation. Examples: walking or jogging on a treadmill, riding a stationary bike or recumbent bike.
- Exercises to strengthen muscles, especially those important for good posture, and to combat osteoporosis. These include weight-bearing exercises and calisthenics for older men and women.
- Exercises to improve joint mobility and prevent or relieve aches and pains. These consist of static stretching positions that are safe and effective for older and inactive people.

Basic Principles:

- See your doctor.
- Take it slow: start at a low, comfortable level and progress gradually.
- Know your limit: learn self-testing methods and stay within your target heart rate zone (see chapter 4).
- Exercise regularly: three to five times per week—Don't make excuses not to exercise!
- Exercise at a heart rate within 50 percent to 85 percent of your capacity.
- Always warm up and cool down: to protect muscles, ligaments, joints, and control blood flow. Muscles need to be warmed up before being thrown into action.
- Don't head for the shower or sauna immediately; this opens up circulation, just as activity does. Wait five to ten minutes!

- Don't compete—except with yourself! Don't overexert yourself to keep up with someone else. Overdoing it stimulates adrenaline, which makes the heart work less efficiently.
- Don't exercise when you're sick with a *fever.* When you're sick, your system is facing one type of challenge. If you double the challenge with exercise, it can be too much. You won't derive many benefits by exercising when you're ill. You might even delay recovery.
- Stretching after a five-to-ten-minute warm-up is of primary importance to fifty-plusers. Stretching improves flexibility and range of motion, and flexibility is one of the first things to be lost with age. As we age, our daily activities don't require us to put all of our muscles and joints through a full range of motion. This causes muscles to shorten and the joints react like rusty hinges.
- Strength plus flexibility in the proper timing and intensity yields coordination.
- Two things to *never* do: work through pain or work for the burn. Pain is a warning. It means you are injuring yourself. PAIN = STOP.
- The keys to getting in shape are determination and consistency. As soon as your body responds and you begin to feel new waves of energy, you'll actually enjoy your exercise program and want to stay in shape.

Some Additional Dos and Don'ts:

- Unless your doctor has prescribed it for you, don't wear a girdle when you exercise; it impairs circulation.
- Don't wear rubber garters to hold up socks or stockings. Don't wear tight-fitting clothing. Keep your body free from restrictions.

- Wear light, loose-fitting clothing: comfortable cotton T-shirt, sports bra, stretch pants/shorts.

Once you get in shape, you can take up a sport. If you walk, join a walking club. If you ride a stationary bike, join a biking club. If you use the rowing machine, go on a canoe trip. If you use a ski machine, go skiing. Enjoy your enhanced balance, coordination, agility, posture, and rhythm—take advantage of it!

EXERCISE AND PREGNANCY

There is probably no other time in a woman's life when fitness is so important as during the months of pregnancy.

TIP 155

The best time to begin to get into shape is before you become pregnant.

Before Pregnancy Concentrate On:

- Overall aerobic fitness. Aerobic exercises are the best for improving your stamina. If you are aerobically fit before you become pregnant, your doctor will probably let you continue your program throughout much of your pregnancy.

- Pelvic fitness. Work up to the highest level of pelvic fitness that you can. Pay particular attention to the strength of your lower back, which will bear a great deal of the stress of your pregnancy.
- Breathing and relaxation. Perform some type of relaxation exercise once a day (i.e. deep abdominal breathing).

During Pregnancy:

- Maintain your cardiovascular program as long as your doctor permits. Sustained aerobic activity should be limited to fifteen minutes, and your pulse should not exceed 140 beats per minute.
- Continue exercises for pelvic fitness. However, exercise in the supine position should be avoided after the fourth month.
- Take care of your back. Relax your back whenever you can; take frequent rest breaks (curling up on your side). As the baby grows, your entire center of gravity shifts. Your posture will change as the natural curve of your back becomes exaggerated. Strong abdominals will help carry the load.
- Do relaxation exercises. You can learn them in a class that teaches exercises and preparation for childbirth.
- If you have not been exercising before you were pregnant, *do not* start now. Start after you've given birth.

After Delivery:

- Right away (hours after the birth) start isometric contractions for the abdomen (if no physical constraints from birth).

- Resume exercise when it's comfortable for you (usually four to six weeks after you give birth).

Warnings:

- Exercise during pregnancy only if your pregnancy is normal and without complications.
- Check with your obstetrician before exercising during pregnancy, to make sure it's okay.
- Danger signs while you're pregnant:
  Pain
  Bleeding
  Rupture of membranes (water breaking)
  Absence of fetal movement

Always:

- Listen to your body
- Avoid fatigue and excessive heat. Core body temperature should be below 101°F. Watch for overheating.
- Make sure you are sufficiently hydrated.
- Engage in static stretching only.
- If problems arise, stop exercising, and see your obstetrician.

TIP 156

If you have not been exercising prior to your pregnancy, do not start an exercise program while

you are pregnant without medical supervision.

When you start an exercise program, your body goes through a tremendous amount of physical and chemical changes, and some of the changes might be harmful to you and your baby-to-be. If you feel like being somewhat active, I recommend doing some light stationary biking with little or no resistance and moderate rpm (40–60).

In conclusion, the more fit you are before you become pregnant, the better chances you'll have for a smoother birth and for having a healthier and stronger child. Giving birth is no easy chore, so you need every advantage you can get. Additionally, if your self-esteem is low during pregnancy because you're not as fit as you can be, you are more apt to become severely depressed from time to time. When you're fit, you feel that you can conquer the world.

I know that there are a number of groups that I have not mentioned; however, I've covered the ones that I'm most frequently asked questions about in my profession. This does not, by any means, represent all of the special population groups, nor does it mean that I do not feel strongly about the importance of fitness for people with osteoporosis, chronic fatigue syndrome, multiple sclerosis, cerebral palsy, and all the other conditions that afflict millions of people each day. I could easily write a book just on special populations. If you have a question on how to improve your fitness level, please do not hesitate to write to me (my address is at the end of the book).

Ten

THE ULTIMATE WORKOUT

If you follow the exercise routine that you're about to read, you will achieve ultimate fitness. It is an exercise program that children can do and teenagers can perform, one that adults, professional athletes, and most of the elderly can also engage in. I call it the ultimate workout because that's exactly what it is—final and conclusive.

This workout is universal. It is designed for thirty to forty-five minutes, and as you get in better shape, you can work up to an hour. If you cannot do a specific exercise because of a medical problem, skip it or replace it with another exercise (which is described) instead of the regular prescribed one.

If you want to replace the bike with a treadmill or a skier, or any other piece of cardiovascular equipment, you may do so. But I highly recommend using a stationary bike if you want the maximum benefits from this workout. Also, if you cannot jump rope because of a medical or orthopedic problem, substitute it with the bike for three to five minutes at 70–90 rpm, or your favorite piece of cardiovascular equipment. Remember to follow the workout exactly as prescribed, and do not skip an exercise unless it aggravates an injury or puts undue stress on your joints or any other part of your body.

If you can do only a few repetitions of any exercise, that's okay, because with time, you will be able to perform many repetitions as you get in better shape.

This workout will not only change your body in two weeks or less, it will give you discipline that will carry over in every other facet of your life. Good luck and be patient. And remember, technique is everything!

Reminder: Get your doctor's approval before performing these or any exercises.

PHASE I: THE WARM-UP

Begin all your workouts with easy-paced aerobic exercises that do not require extremes in movement. Light jogging, walking in place, or biking actually increases circulation through the muscles, raises heart rate, and warms up the cardiovascular system. Warm up for 6 to 10 minutes.

PHASE II: STRETCHING

- Always use a static stretch, holding stretch for 15 to 30 seconds.
- Never bounce while stretching.
- Do not hold your breath while stretching.

A. Arm circles: With arms outstretched, slowly pull arms backward, which will stretch out the chest and shoulder muscles. By pulling your fingers and wrist backward, the front of the upper arm and forearms will also effectively be stretched. Slowly circle your arms in a clockwise direction for 5 revolutions and then for 5 revolutions in the counterclockwise direction.

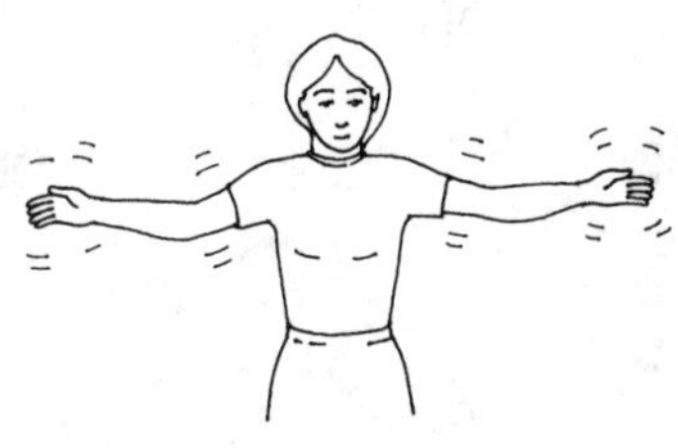

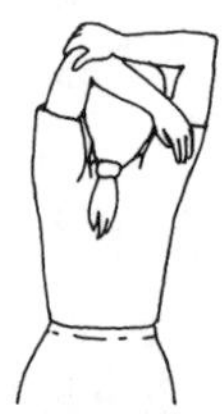

B. Triceps: With arms overhead, gently pull the left elbow behind your head with the right hand. Hold when you reach a comfortable stretch in the rear shoulder and upper back. Switch arms and repeat.

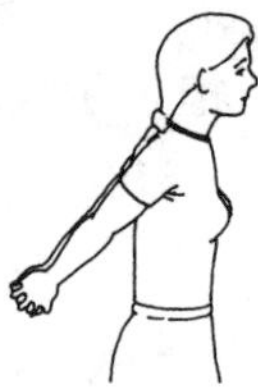

C. Upper back and chest: Grasp hands behind your back, then lift arms up and hold until you feel a good stretch in the chest, front shoulder, and front of upper arm.

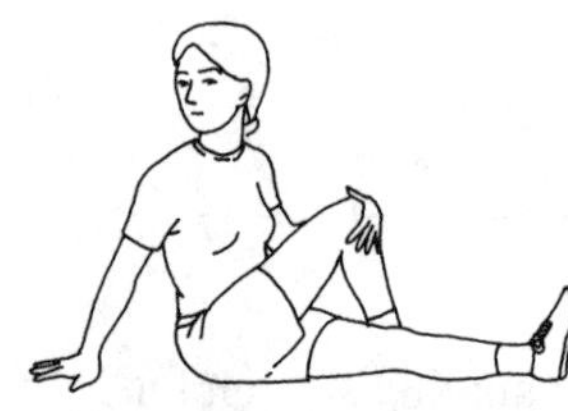

D. Spine twist: Keeping the left leg straight, right arm behind for support, cross right leg over and place foot outside the left knee. With the left hand or elbow on the right knee, slowly turn your head and look over your right shoulder while simultaneously pulling the knee in the opposite direction; hold. You will feel pressure in the hip, side, and upper back. Repeat on opposite side.

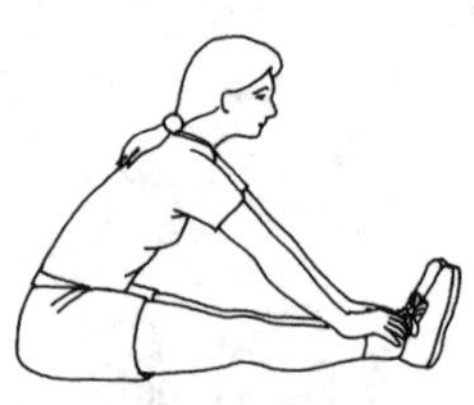

E. Hamstring: With legs straight and ankles flexed, bend forward from the hips and reach out toward the toes, holding the stretch. You will feel tightness just behind the knee, in the upper calf, and in the lower back area.

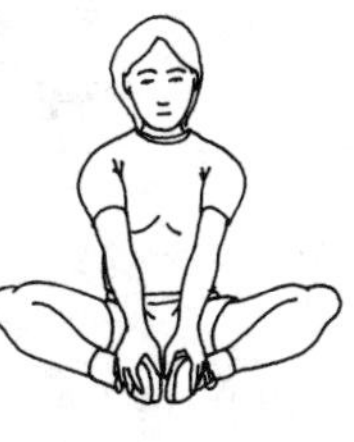

F. Groin: In sitting position, put soles of feet together; grab and hold your ankles. Gently pull heels toward groin area. For a nice and relaxed inner thigh stretch simply let your knees relax down toward the floor. Lean upper body slightly forward and press out against your knees with your elbows to increase stretch.

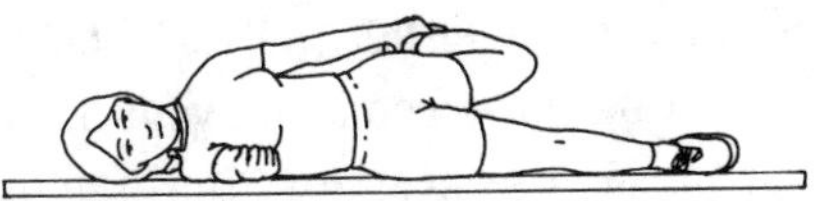

G. Quadriceps: While lying on your side, pull top leg back by grasping front of the ankle. Gently pull heel back and up behind buttocks. Repeat on opposite side.

H. Calf: Stand away from the wall or solid support and lean on it with hands placed against the wall. Place one leg forward in a flexed position; back leg is straight. Lean toward wall while holding the stretch. Repeat, stretching the other leg.

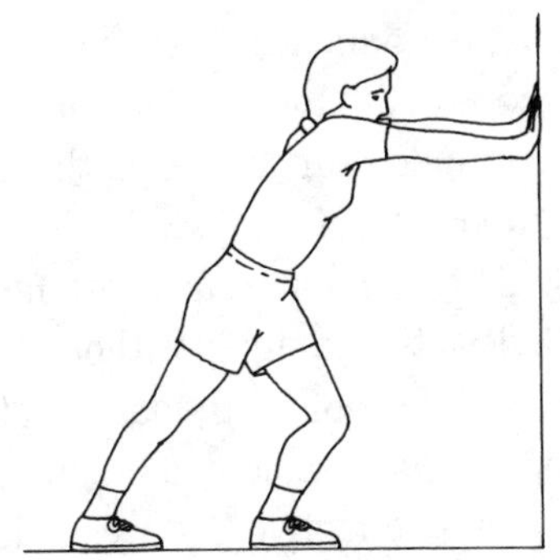

Important Things to Remember:

- All exercises that require you to be on the ground should be performed *only* on an exercise mat.
- When choosing to use either the 10-lb. curl bar or 15-lb. straight bar be sure to consider your body type first.
- Check your pulse after every two to three exercises to ensure that you're in your zone.
- Sidebenders are used for active rest and to tighten the sides of your stomach.
- If you feel that this workout is not challenging enough, perform each set of exercises twice.

How to Jump Rope:

1. Practice swinging rope over head without jumping.
2. Jump just high enough for rope to pass under feet (1–1.5 inches off the ground). Jump with both feet at once. Jumping higher than two inches will create unnecessary stress on the legs, increasing the potential for injury.
3. Move wrists in time with feet.
4. Practice jumping without rope in hands. When comfortable with movement, try it with the rope.
5. *Caution:* Avoid double jumping; your workout will not be as effective. After each jump the rope should pass under your feet.

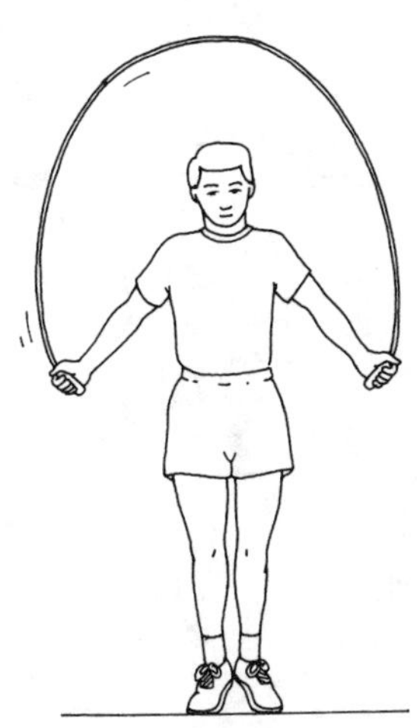

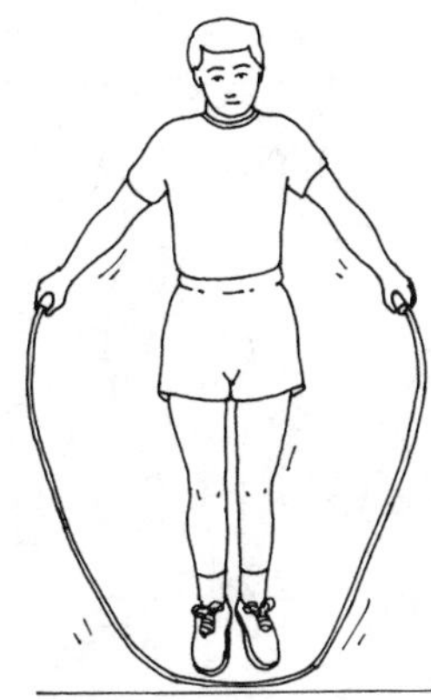

1. Do one set (50–200) of jump rope repetitions.

Rest after jumping rope by doing sidebenders until you catch your breath (1–2 minutes).

Sidebenders: Rest an aerobic bar or broomstick across your shoulders and slowly bend your upper body from side to side. Do not stop in the middle, and keep at a slow, steady pace. Keep chest lifted and head up.

Do 20–40 sidebenders.

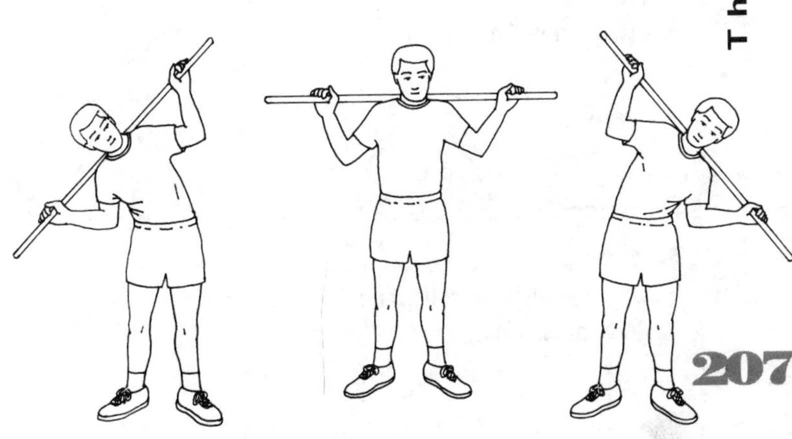

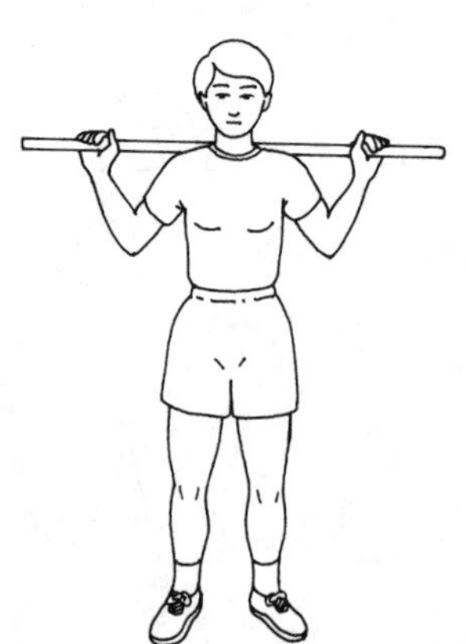

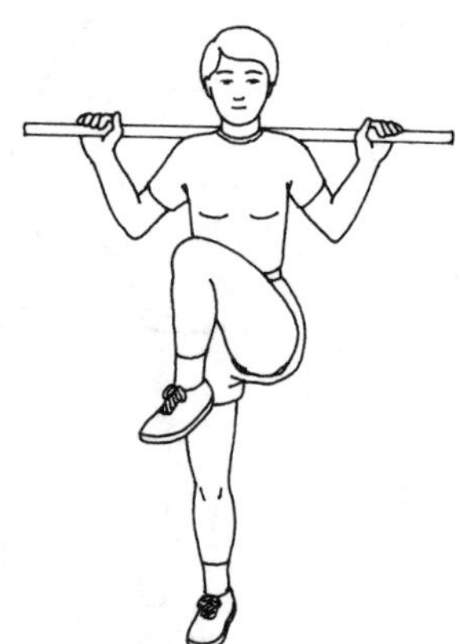

2. Standing Knee to Opposite Chest

1. Hold the bar behind your head and rest on shoulders. Feet and hands are at least shoulder-width apart with soft knees.
2. Bring left knee up toward right shoulder, keeping back straight and abdominals contracted. Bring foot back to starting position.
3. Do not transfer weight to other leg when returning; keep weight on straight leg at all times.
4. Repeat 25–50 times at a steady pace.
5. Switch legs and repeat.

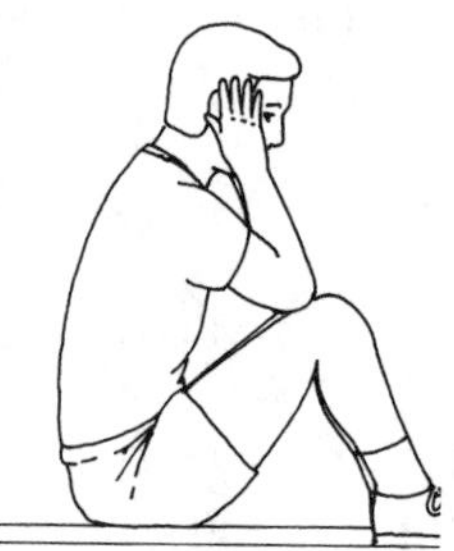

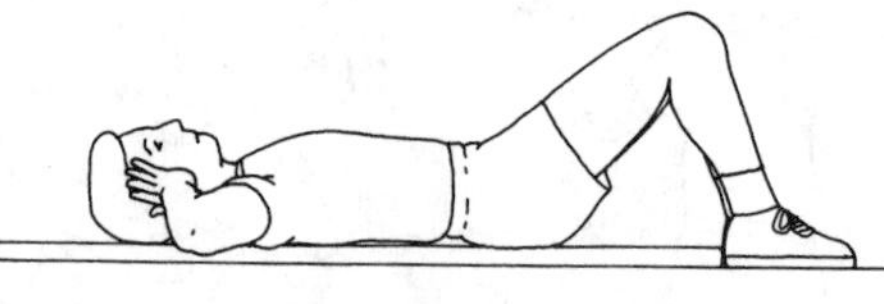

3. Sit-ups

1. Lie on your back, with knees bent, feet flat on the floor, heels up against the mat.

2. Place fingertips on your temples, palms facing in, elbows out. Contract your abs, and leading with your chest slowly curl all the way up, closing elbows.
3. Elbows should touch your knees, exhale upon sitting up.
4. Curl down and repeat.
5. Do 20–50 full bent-knee sit-ups, progressing up to 100.

4. Leg-outs

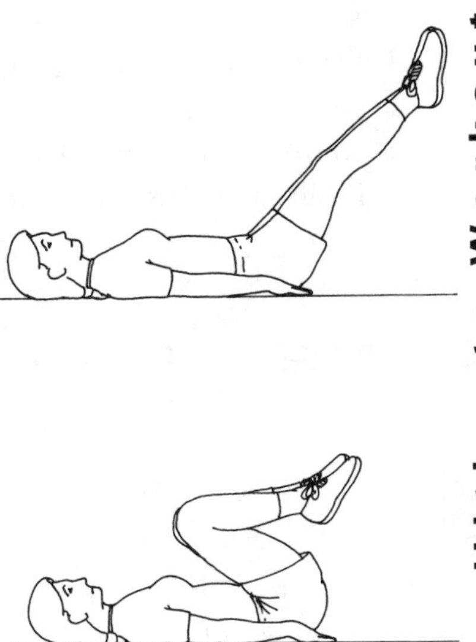

1. Lying on your back, with hands under buttocks, palms down, pull knees into chest.
2. Slowly straighten legs out with toes pointed to six inches from the ground (higher if your back aches at all).
3. Inhale while pulling knees toward chest; exhale as you straighten legs.
4. Repeat 15–30 times, progressing up to 100.

5. Second set of jump rope (50–200) followed by sidebenders.

6. 10-lb. Curl Bar or 15-lb. Straight Bar Routine

A. Push-Outs

1. Feet shoulder-width apart for correct balance.
2. Hold bar at shoulder-width grip and rest on top of chest. Make sure back is straight and knees are slightly flexed.
3. Extend arms straight out and exhale while doing so.
4. Let the bar drop to front of thighs and roll up to starting position, while inhaling.
5. Do 10–20 repetitions (build up to 50).

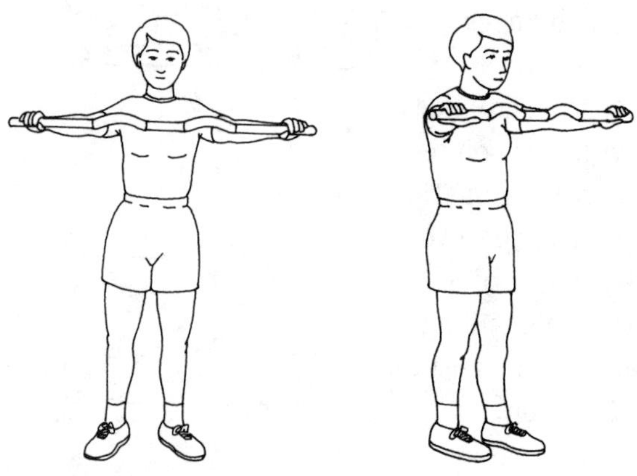

B. Behind-the-Neck Press

1. Feet at least shoulder-width apart.
2. Hold bar at shoulder-width grip behind neck and rest on back of shoulders.
3. Extend arms upward and exhale.

4. Bend arms until bar touches back of shoulders while inhaling.
5. Do 10–20 repetitions (build up to 50).

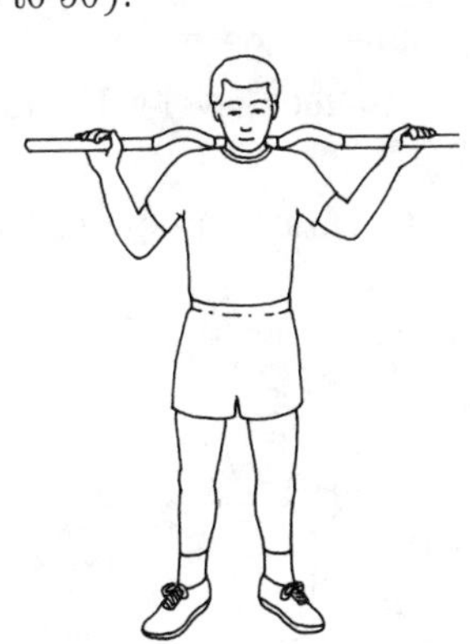

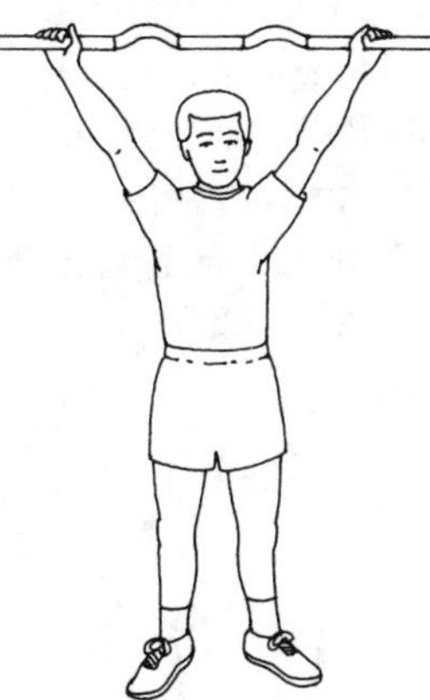

C. Front Press

1. Feet at least shoulder-width apart.
2. Hold bar at shoulder-width grip and rest on top of chest.
3. Push straight upward and exhale.
4. Bend arms and let bar down to chest while inhaling.
5. Do 10–20 repetitions (build up to 50).

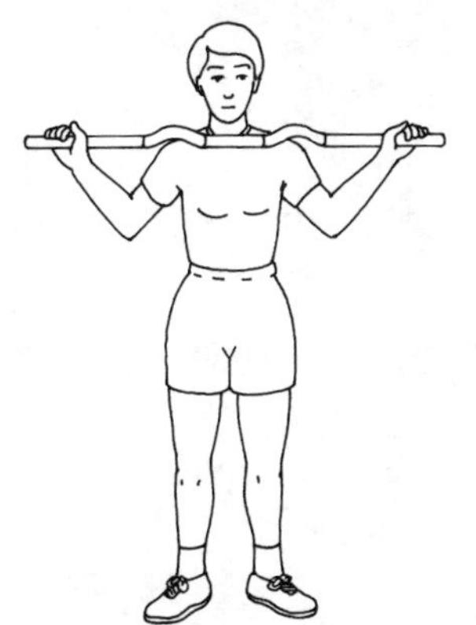

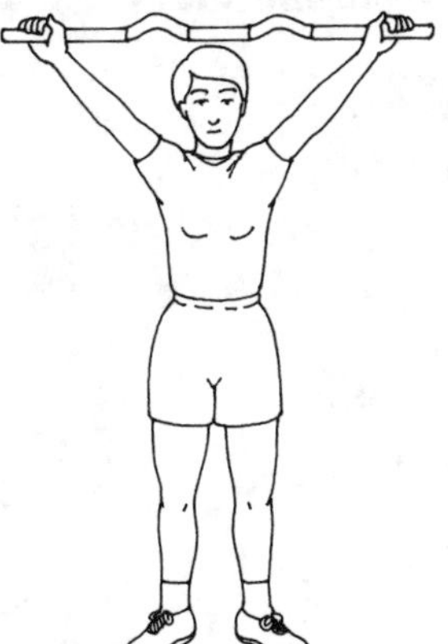

D. Upright Rows

1. Feet at least shoulder-width apart.
2. Hold bar with narrow grip with hands 4–6 inches apart and arms fully extended below waist.
3. Pull upward and bring bar to neck level with elbows out above the bar; exhale.
4. Bring bar down to starting position while inhaling.
5. Do 10–20 repetitions (build up to 50).

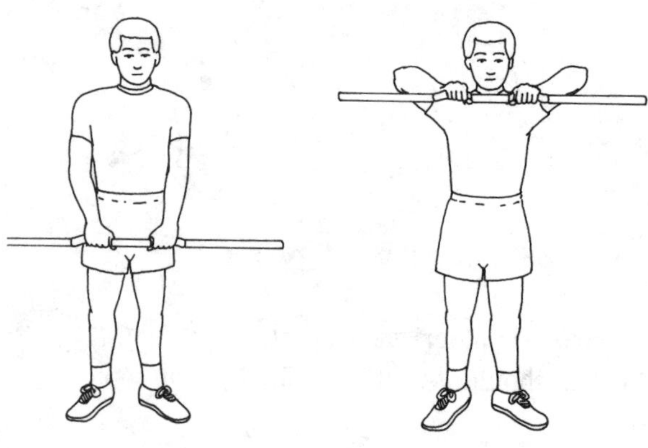

7. Third set of jump rope (50–200) followed by sidebenders.

8. Crunch

1. Lie on your back with knees bent forward as illustrated.
2. With hands clasped at base of neck, bring elbows in and crunch up, touching elbows to knees, exhaling.
3. Return to starting position, inhaling.
4. Repeat 15–30 times (build up to 100).

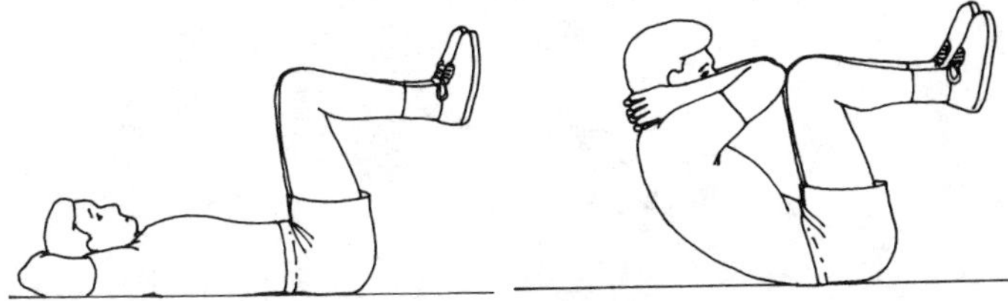

9. V-Scissors

1. Lying on your back with your hands holding sides of mat, raise your legs to a ninety-degree angle (as you strengthen you can go lower, but never less than forty-five degrees).
2. Keep the small of your back on the floor and open legs as wide apart as possible. Bring legs together with toes pointed.
3. Repeat 20–40 repetitions (build up to 100).

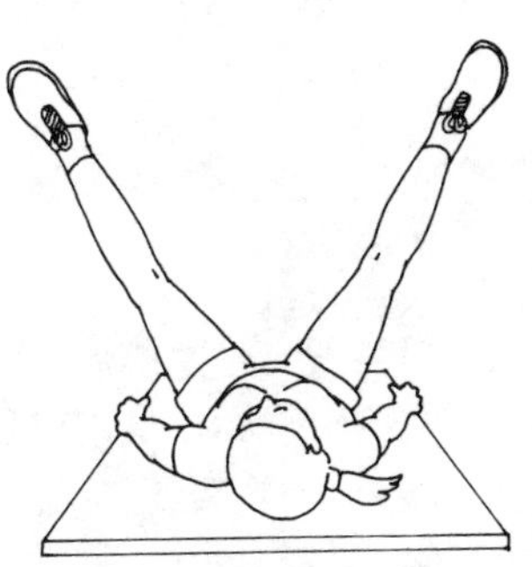

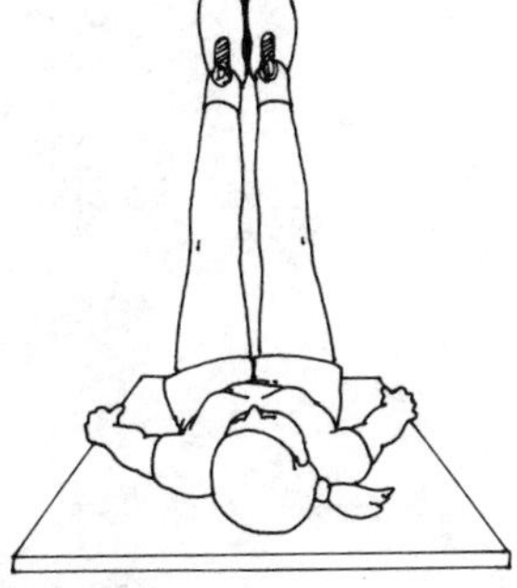

10. Push-ups

1. On hands and toes (advanced).
   On hands and knees with ankles crossed (basic).
2. Point fingers forward and place hands shoulder-width apart. Keep abdominals contracted and lower chest as close to the floor as possible, then slowly push up.
3. Exhale while pushing up, inhale going down.
4. Repeat 10–20 times (build up to 100).

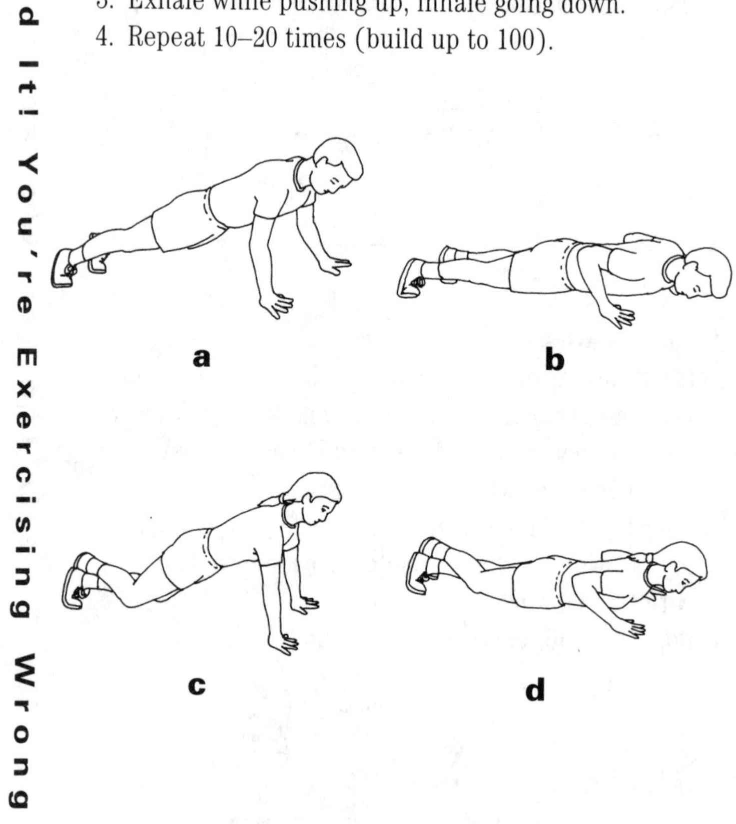

11. Tricep Push-ups

1. On all fours (see push-ups), place hands close together on the floor with fingertips angled slightly in, so index Fingers and thumbs form a triangle.
2. Lower chest as close to the floor as possible, then slowly push up.
3. Exhale while pushing up; inhale going down.
4. Repeat 5–15 times (build to 50).

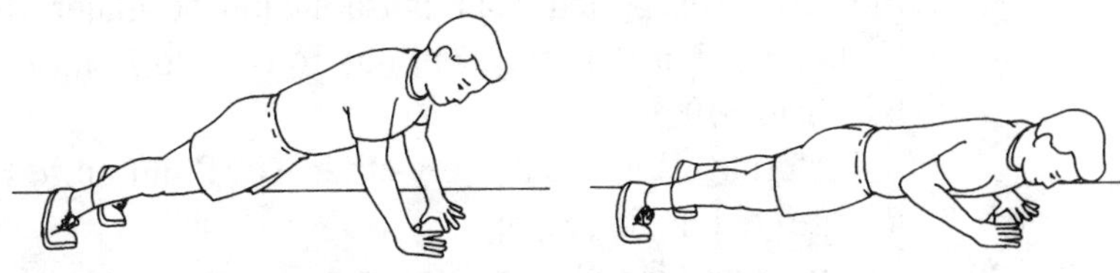

12. Perform 25–50 standing knee to opposite chest (see #2).

13. Chair Dips

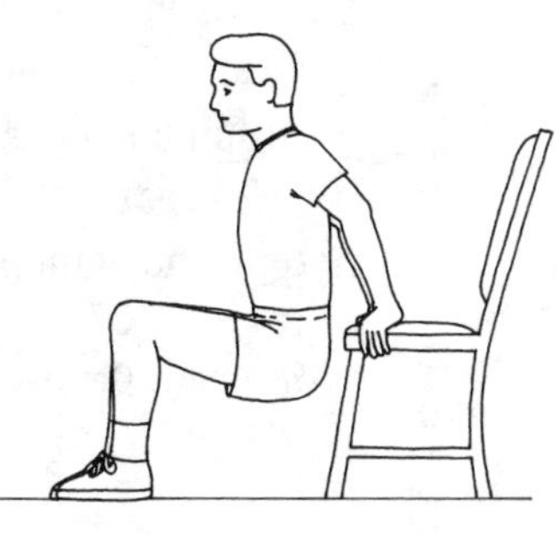

1. Place palms on edge of chair, holding your weight with your arms.
2. Hold on to the seat of a chair with buttocks planted in front of chair and feet planted in front of buttocks, knees bent.
3. Bend arms and slowly lower body; exhale as you push back up.
4. Repeat 7–20 times (build up to 50).

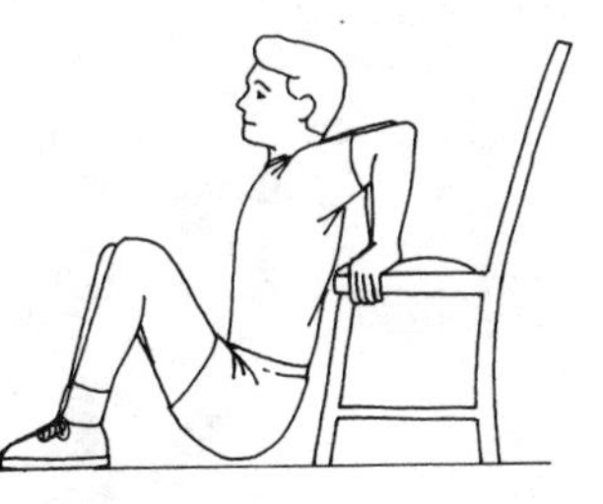

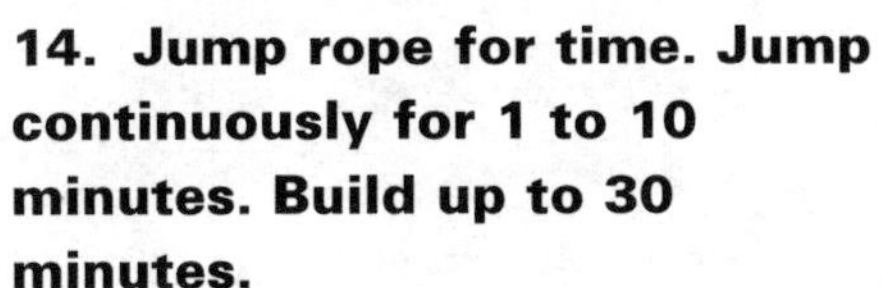

14. Jump rope for time. Jump continuously for 1 to 10 minutes. Build up to 30 minutes.

PHASE IV: COOLDOWN

End *all* your workouts with an easy-paced aerobic exercise. Walk (1.5–3.0 mph) or bike (40–60 rpm) for 3–5 minutes, until breathing has returned to normal.

Check pulse at end of your workout. Five minutes after the cool-down period, your pulse should be under 100 beats per minute. If not, continue to cool down until it falls below 100.

Perform this workout every other day. Build up to 30 minutes of jumping rope.

If your goal is to lose weight: run, jog, stationary bike, or jump rope on the days in between for 20 to 40 minutes and stretch afterward.

If your goal is to firm up and tone: build up to performing all the exercises, except rope jumping, twice within one hour

To reduce hips, legs, and buttocks: do more jumping rope and standing knee to opposite chest.

Reminder: Get your doctor's approval before performing these or any exercises.

Conclusion

The research done for this book was *all* based on practical experience. The impetus for this book came from people like you and me who are searching for a simple fitness routine that we can follow for the rest of our lives, despite common constraints.

This book has been written for those who do not exercise and for those who presently do but are not pleased with the way they look.

I implore you to follow the wisdom and guidance outlined and illustrated in this book. Remember, just because you're exercising, that doesn't mean you're getting fit!

If you have a question concerning a fitness or lifestyle topic, please don't hesitate to contact us.

Program Director
Exude Inc.
16 East 52nd Street, Third Floor
New York, NY 10022
1-800-24-EXUDE or (212) 644-9559
FAX: (212) 759-4387

Index

YES! I WOULD LIKE TO ORDER:

_____ JUMPING TOWARDS FITNESS KIT @ 39.95 EA. ADD $7.00 SHIPPING & HANDLING PER KIT

_____ JUMPING TOWARDS FITNESS, VOL I VIDEO @ 19.95 EA. ADD $5.00 SHIPPING & HANDLING PER VIDEO

_____ JUMP ROPE @ 14.95 EA. ADD $3.00 SHIPPING & HANDLING PER ROPE

_____ JUMPING ROPE PLATFORM @ 99.95 EA. ADD $19.00 SHIPPING & HANDLING PER PLATFORM

_____ AEROBIC BAR @ 33.95 EA. ADD $7.00 SHIPPING & HANDLING PER BAR

_____ HOLD IT! YOU'RE EXERCISING WRONG BOOK @ 9.95 EA. ADD $3.00 SHIPPING & HANDLING PER BOOK

_____ ABDOMINAL/STRETCHING MAT @ 29.95 EA. ADD $7.00 SHIPPING & HANDLING PER MAT

WE ACCEPT MASTERCARD, VISA, AMEX, DISCOVER, CHECK OR MONEY ORDER FOR PAYMENT.

PLEASE MAKE ALL CHECKS PAYABLE TO:

CORE FITNESS MANAGEMENT

IF YOU ARE PAYING BY CREDIT CARD, PLEASE INCLUDE THE FULL NAME ON THE CARD, THE BILLING ADDRESS OF THE CARD, THE CREDIT CARD NUMBER AND CREDIT CARD EXPIRATION DATE FROM THE CREDIT CARD.

PLEASE INCLUDE YOUR NAME, SHIPPING ADDRESS AND PHONE NUMBER WITH AREA CODE SO WE MAY PROPERLY PROCESS YOUR ORDER.

IF YOU ARE PAYING BY CREDIT CARD, YOU CAN FAX YOUR ORDER TO:

516 287-2096

IF YOU ARE MAILING US YOUR ORDER, PLEASE MAIL IT TO:

CORE FITNESS MANAGEMENT
21 LITTLE NECK ROAD
SOUTHAMPTON, NY 11968